your Makeover

UNIVERSE

your Makeover

by MORGEN SCHICK DEMANN

Photographs by BILL WESTMORELAND

simple

ways

for

any

woman

to

look

her

BEST

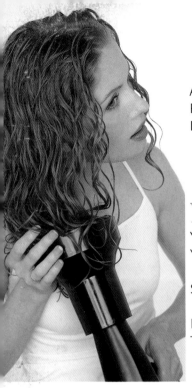

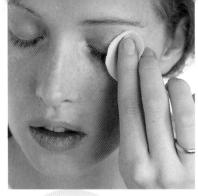

your skin 12

your makeup 42

your hair 10

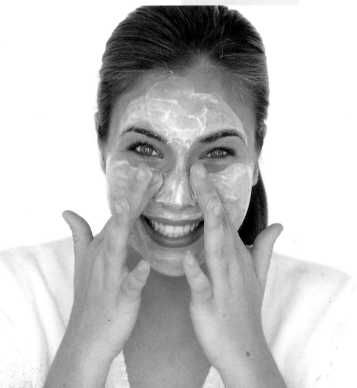

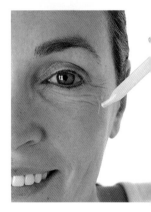

Contents

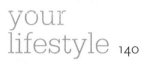

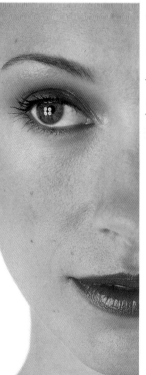

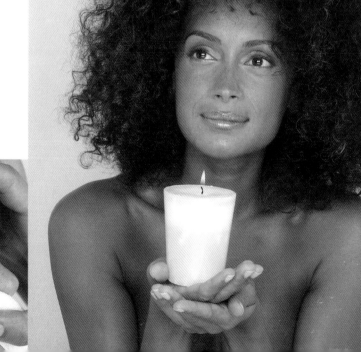

First published in the United
States of America in 2000
by UNIVERSE PUBLISHING
A Division of Rizzoli
International Publications, Inc.
300 Park Avenue South
New York, New York 10010

© by Morgen Schick DeMann

00 01 02 / 10 9 8 7 6 5 4 3 2 1

Designed by Bill Anton |
Service Station

Printed in Malaysia

I dedicate
this book to my
Nanni,
the matriarch
of the most
loving family
a girl
could be
blessed with.

ACKNOWLEDGMENTS

My love and appreciation go to my parents, Donald and Virginia, for their endless support and inspiration; my brothers, Peter and Matthew, whom I adore; my sister, Beth, whose intelligence and beauty amaze me; my auntie, Kathlyn Budde, for being up for a makeover anytime; and my cousins for their humor and support.

This book would not have been possible without the tireless efforts of many people: Bill Westmoreland and Sacha, whose unending talent and commitment made this book what it is; Dr. Edmond Griffin, who patiently answered all my questions; Patricia Tucker-Horne for her help. Special thanks go to my extended family at Ford Models, especially Patty Sicular, a wonderful agent and a very special person, and Katie, Eileen, and Jerry Ford for their constant support and confidence in me. I'm very grateful to Elisabeth Halfpapp from the Lotte Berk Method, whose knowledge and energy are reflected in our exercise section; Julia Labaton, who always provides useful information and samples of new products; Clark Gregory, a supreme colorist and great friend; Christy Chis at Mario Badescu Skin Care for keeping my face camera-ready; Michelle Huh for her wonderful work on the nail section in this book; Kit D'Fever and Independence Pass Productions for all their help and support. I'm grateful to Julie Kofman at Cosmair and Cindi Galiher and Ida Monna at Laura Mercier for providing products for me to test. My heartfelt thanks go to Marita for always believing, Christie for her organizational skills, and Lisa J. Haynes for getting me there.

Very special thanks to the beautiful women whose images grace these pages: Elizabeth Aiken, Alise Allen, Patricia Hartmann-Costantino, Wanda Geddie Brickner, Christie Forstmann, Brenda Schad, Marita Stavrou, Sarah Stavrou, Beth Schick, Nanou Caillet, Sophie Hirtzel, Kedaki Lipton, Jillian Johnson, Lisa Shaub, Gloria Barnes, Marie St. Victor,

Andrea Bundonis, Jana Schoep, Audra Marie, Susana Esteban, Caroline Grasso, Julia Labaton, and Melanie Woods.

Thanks to Alex Tart at Universe Publishing for loving this book even though she's a little "makeup challenged"; Charles Miers, Bonnie Eldon, Scott Lavelle, and Belinda Hellinger at Universe for all their help; Bill Anton at Service Station for making the book as beautiful as it is user-friendly; Noah Lukeman of Lukeman Literary Management, without whom this book truly would never have happened. I can't thank you enough for finding me.

To Larry, Gloria, Todd, and Rosemary DeMann, thank you for being my East Coast family.

And finally, to my husband, Drew. For a cerebral, analytical man he can spot a bad dye job or an overly lined lip from a mile away now. Your love, support, humor, and patience are inspirational. I love you.

FOREWORD

BY ELEEN FORD AND KATIE FORD

We are especially pleased to be able to contribute to this remarkable book, for in it Morgen Schick DeMann has taken her experience as a model and makeup artist and has endeavored to share it with women everywhere in the form of practical, real-life advice. It gets to the core of what most women seek: simple, healthy, and inexpensive beauty solutions for an active lifestyle.

Experience is one thing Morgen possesses in abundance. Over the past decade at Ford, Morgen's commitment to her career has never wavered, nor has her enthusiasm for finding innovative and simple beauty solutions—ones that serve her just as well in private life as they do under the burning lights of a photo shoot. Endowed with an innate sense of style and a straightforward approach to beauty, Morgen is a modeling agent's dream: flexible yet attentive to detail, focused yet prepared for the unexpected, naturally confident yet thoughtful of those around her.

And if Morgen's success outside of Ford (as spokesperson for a cosmetics line and a TV commentator, for example) is any indication, her talents are as diverse as they are strong.

It is precisely this diversity, this flexibility and natural flair, that Morgen brings to *Your Makeover*. The book is comprehensive but not overwhelming, with easy-to-navigate chapters that guide women around the pitfalls of skin, hair, and body care toward accessible formulas that virtually any woman can benefit from. Yet Morgen is a perfectionist at heart, and her regimens, while not overly complex, are sensitive to the fact that all women are different, physically and emotionally. To any woman who opens this book, however, Morgen's message is clear: Every woman possesses her own unique beauty, and every woman deserves the chance to look her best.

Eileen is the founder of Ford Models. Eileen's daughter, Katie, is now CEO.

In my last eleven years as a Ford model, I have worked with some of the top hairstylists and makeup artists in the world. I have witnessed remarkable makeovers on hundreds of women and have come away with one conclusion: <u>anyone can look fabulous</u>. If you use what the experts use, learn why they choose one product over another, and learn the correct application techniques, you can make it happen.

Most models, swamped by hairstylists, makeup artists, manicurists, and photographers, don't pay attention to what's being done to them. But I always did. As a professional whose livelihood it is to look beautiful all the time, whether there was a crew of stylists with me or not, I felt I should be able to do my own hair and makeup as well as anyone else could. So I learned how to give myself a makeover in every situation: various lighting conditions, different times of the month, unexpected weather. I learned how to deal with every beauty emergency under the sun, from sunburn to acne to dry, peeling skin. I researched every aspect of the beauty and fashion industries, from facials to concealers to hair conditioners to how to buy designer clothing at a discount no matter where you live. Over time, I began doing makeovers on family, friends, and anyone I could get my hands on. I did makeup on other models for their portfolios. I even did their weddings.

I realized that there is no woman out there—even among supermodels—who cannot always look better. In this book I will share all the secrets and tips I've learned the hard way over the last eleven years, and I'll teach you how to fix all the flaws you thought could never be fixed. Whether it's the five-minute makeover for the woman on the run—the fuller lip, the more sensuous eye, the more prominent cheekbone—or the complete makeover, incorporating full body changes in nutrition, exercise, hair, and dress, this book will speak to every woman out there. I've chosen women of all ages, races, skin types, and

INTRODUCTION

backgrounds for the pictures in this book, with the hope that every woman will be able to find someone who reminds her of herself. I've tried to cut through the mystery surrounding the modeling business, to show you practical ideas that any woman can learn, apply, and enjoy. I've seen hundreds of makeovers throughout the years, and I always felt as though the women looked overly made-up. I also didn't think they would be able to replicate the makeup on their own. I wanted to show easy practical tips that I'm sure you'll be able to do without me there.

If you wonder why most of the women in magazines and beauty books look as though their skin and hair are perfect, it is probably because the images have been retouched. In other words, the flaws were removed from the photos by hand or with a computer program. I've always thought that this is a disservice to women, because as hard as they studied a makeup book, and as conscientiously as they used what the experts use, they might never attain what they see in a magazine. I wanted you to be able to see that all of the secrets in this book are attainable for you, for real, so we didn't retouch the photographs in this book. What you see here is exactly what we did. I want you to know that I understand and have experienced much of what you've felt about your body, face, hair, and your overall health and appearance. Maybe I was blessed with a certain bone structure but I wasn't blessed with perfect skin, hair, nails, or metabolism. All of this I've had to fine-tune on my own. I've had to learn how to enhance and maintain every aspect of my body.

I don't think that everyone looks better with makeup; or that giving yourself a makeover means there's something wrong with the way you look. It simply means that you want the option to change your look, bring out certain features, or downplay those that bother you. Always cherish what you have, and keep an open mind.

your skin

Your skin is your most important asset. It is the canvas on which a makeup artist can begin; if your skin is problematic, it doesn't much matter what eye shadow you have on. So the skin is the first thing we'll look at in this book.

Anyone will tell you that water is the most important ingredient for great skin. It's true. <u>Drink liters of water every day</u>. Other things are important, too. <u>Don't pick at your skin</u>. <u>Don't play with your face—ever</u>. Sit on your hands if you have to. The oil, dirt, and bacteria on your fingers should never come into contact with the delicate skin on your face. Be conscious of the objects that touch your skin throughout the day: the phone, your hair, pens resting on your cheek or chin. The bacteria on all of these items could cause breakouts if you have sensitive skin. As a model I have artists layering all different brands and types of makeup on my face every day. I don't have the luxury of asking what the expiration dates of the products are or whether they last washed their brushes and sponges in this century. I can usually tell if I will have a bad reaction or not within a few minutes. I also don't have the time to recover from terrible

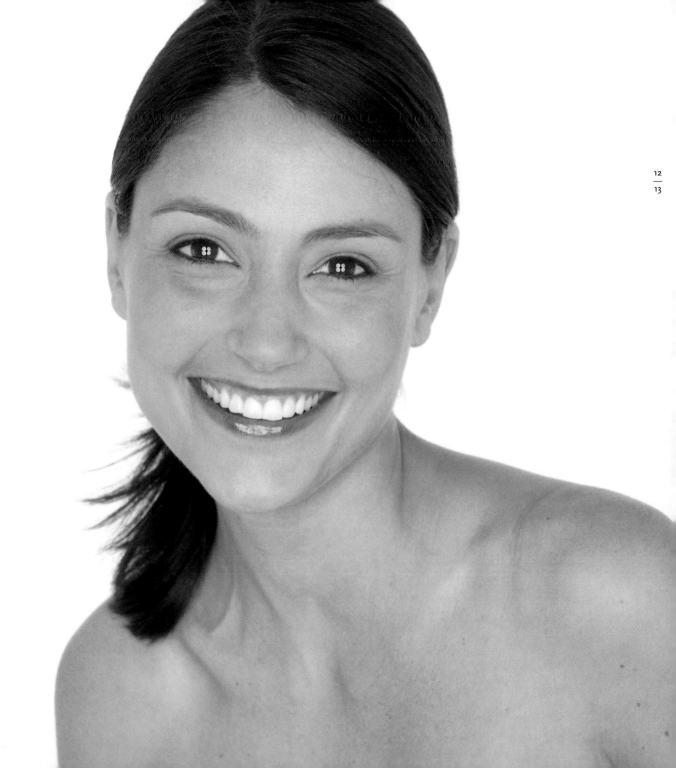

breakouts so I have to know which products will prevent bad makeup from affecting my skin before it happens.

Most dermatologists say that what you eat will affect the condition of your skin. Some foods I eat definitely cause my breakouts. The usual suspects like chocolate and ice cream don't seem to bother me, but licorice and vodka make me break out. If you try to remember what you have eaten just before your skin breaks out, you should be able to figure out what doesn't sit well with your system. There are allergy tests that you can take, but they are expensive. If you seem to break out all the time and the dermatologist often has to prescribe medicine for you, definitely look into getting tested.

Changes in hormones can also affect your skin. You can't prevent these, but a healthy skin-care routine will help minimize the breakouts and other problems they can cause.

your skin type

Let's take an objective look at your face. Place yourself in front of a mirror that has a magnifying effect and turn on as bright a light as you can. We need to see the truth. Look closely at your face from forehead to chin, including under your jawbone and neck. Notice that you have different sized pores on different parts of your face. Notice that you have almost no pores around your eyes. Keep this in mind when you're thinking about moisture. Only where the skin has pores can it absorb and retain moisture. That's why we see signs of aging around the eyes first: there's nothing to keep moisture and collagen in.

I never understand why companies make products designed for skin that is dry, normal, oily, or combination. In my opinion, **everyone has combination skin**. Most of us actually have each type of skin somewhere on our face. Look at your face and chart out where each area is.

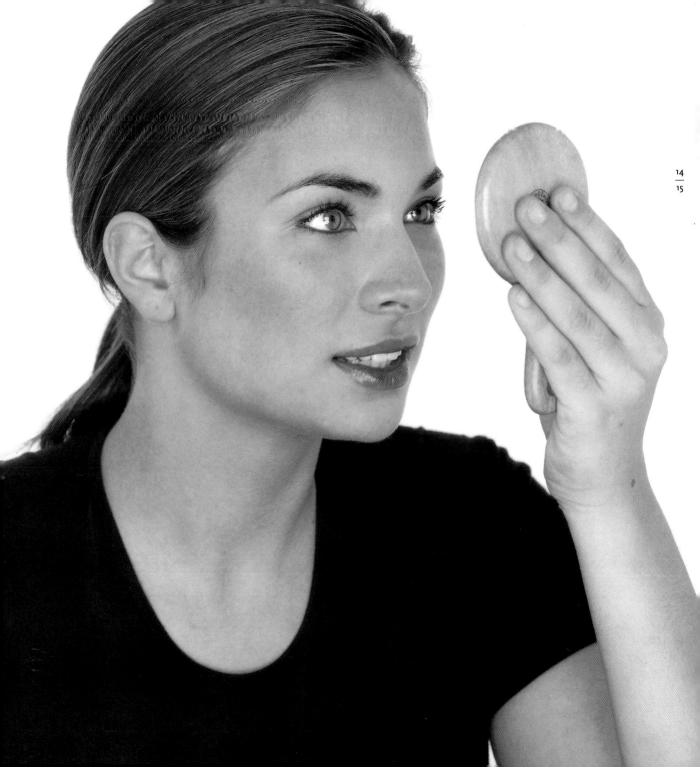

Start at your hairline. Is it flaky? That would make it dry at the scalp and hairline.

Now look at your forehead. Is it usually shiny only a few hours after you wash? If you also have some slight lines across your forehead, don't rule out oily—it just means that you may express yourself by lifting your eyebrows and with time you have developed some lines. We will discuss options for those lines later on. If you never get shiny on your forehead then your skin there is normal to dry.

Move to the area that most people call the T-zone. I find the area between my eyes and down my nose is the oiliest part of my face. On your face determine what that strip is for you.

Now move to your cheekbone and hollow, which should be treated as two different places. Most women have more moisture on the temple and cheekbone than in the hollow. I get many of my pimples on the cheekbone because it's the part I touch with my hands or with blush and a brush. My cheek hollow is usually drier.

Now look at the area around your mouth. Do you have pimples around your lip line? How about under your lower lip? That little crevice under your lip is a perfect place for bacteria, especially if you touch your chin with the phone receiver. The same goes for the jaw line. We lean our chins on our hands or cradle the phone on our shoulder when we need to keep our hands free. Try to hold the phone with your hands only or keep some alcohol wipes around to clean it often.

Once you've identified the different skin types on your face, you can begin to clean, deep cleanse, and moisturize.

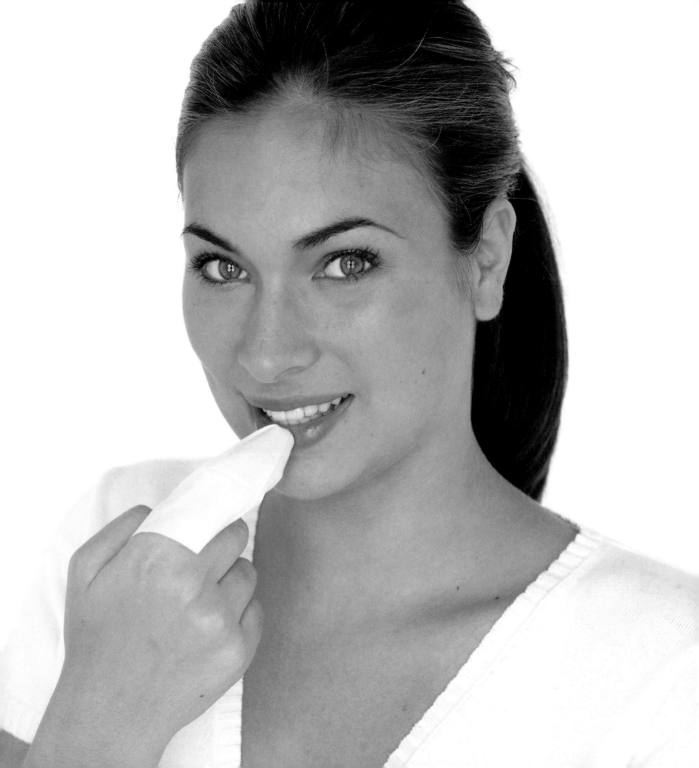

your daily
skin-care routine

Makeup Removal

Your makeup remover should be selected according to your makeup and skin routine. If you use waterproof mascara, you need a heavier oil-based remover. If you wear very little makeup then a mild remover/cleanser will do. It's important to select the right makeup remover so you don't need to rub aggressively in order to get the skin clean. If your makeup needs to be vigorously rubbed off and your eyelashes seem to be falling out, the remover you're using doesn't work. I actually use one for my face and a separate product for my eyes. Cosmetic companies now make disposable makeup removal wipes, which are great when you're traveling.

First, completely saturate the eye area. Let the remover do its job before you start wiping it off.

Swipe the eye area from the inside out. Never rub hard on your eyes. A few seconds is all it takes.

Gently wipe from the nose to the temple. Never pull the skin. <u>You must always be gentle when touching your skin with your fingers</u>. Stretching that delicate tissue is a sure way to get sagging skin.

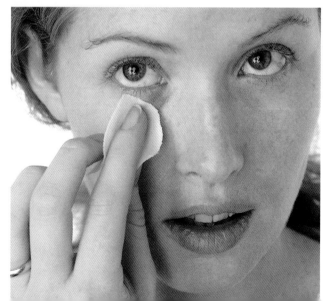

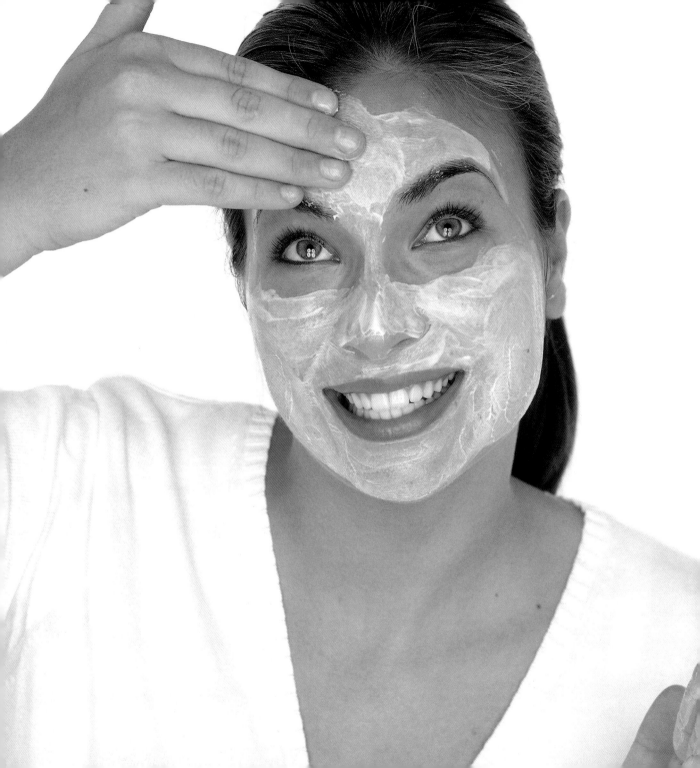

CLEANSING

Once you have taken your makeup off, you should use a pH-balanced gentle cleanser that has no perfume or alcohol. Your skin has to battle many foreign substances already, so keep cleansers as pure as you can get them. I use them all over and really massage them into my skin.

Once your skin is clean make sure you rinse with warm water, not hot. You don't need to scald your delicate skin to make sure it's clean. I have friends who only wash their face with bottled water and swear that it's the secret to perfect skin. I've never done it, but it may be worth a try if you can afford it.

After cleansing, your face should feel clean but still supple. If it feels like you just sucked every drop of moisture out of it, your face will have to work overtime to replace that moisture, and if your skin is oily it actually overproduces sebum and you end up where you started.

If your skin is dry, you may want to try a cream-based cleanser that is simply wiped off with a damp towel. My Nanni (grand-mother in Italian) has dry skin and uses a cold cream, never soap. At ninety years old, she has skin like a baby's.

BRUSH THOSE LIPS!

This may sound strange, but every night after I brush my teeth, but before I rinse, I brush my lips with my toothbrush. This is an easy and inexpensive way to keep your lips supple and to clear off any dead skin. Remember to brush lightly so you don't scrape your lips and put on some lip balm when you're finished. I promise that after the first night your lips will already feel smooth and soft.

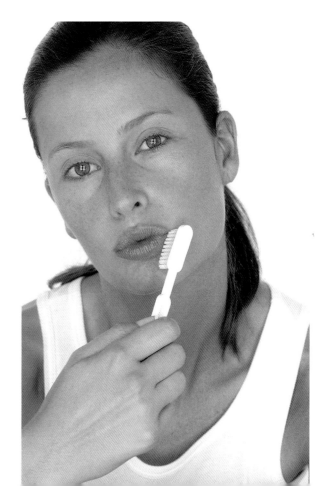

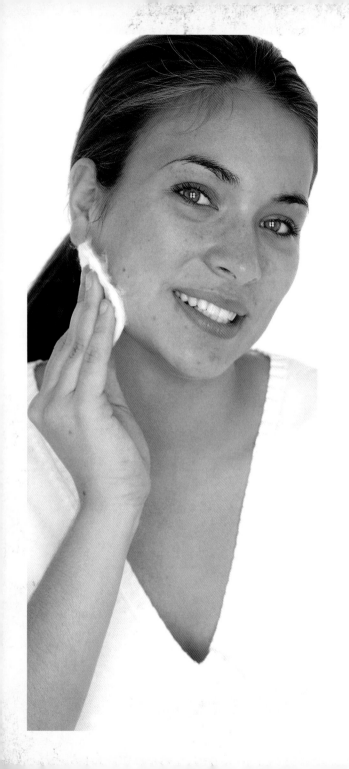

TONERS

Some dermatologists recommend toners to balance your skin's pH after washing. I believe that if your cleanser is correct you won't need this additional step. But if you have oily skin or you love the squeaky-clean feeling of a toner, just be sure you find one that has no alcohol (those can be stripping, and you'll just have to rehydrate your skin after using them). Remember to apply toner only where your skin gets oily—usually in the T-zone and around the mouth.

HYDRATION

I have several moisturizers in my cabinet. I use an oil-free moisturizer with a high SPF in the spring and summer and a heavier moisturizer with a lower SPF in the fall and winter. At night I use a heavier cream that contains alpha hydroxy. I know this sounds complicated but when you're doing it every day it becomes second nature.

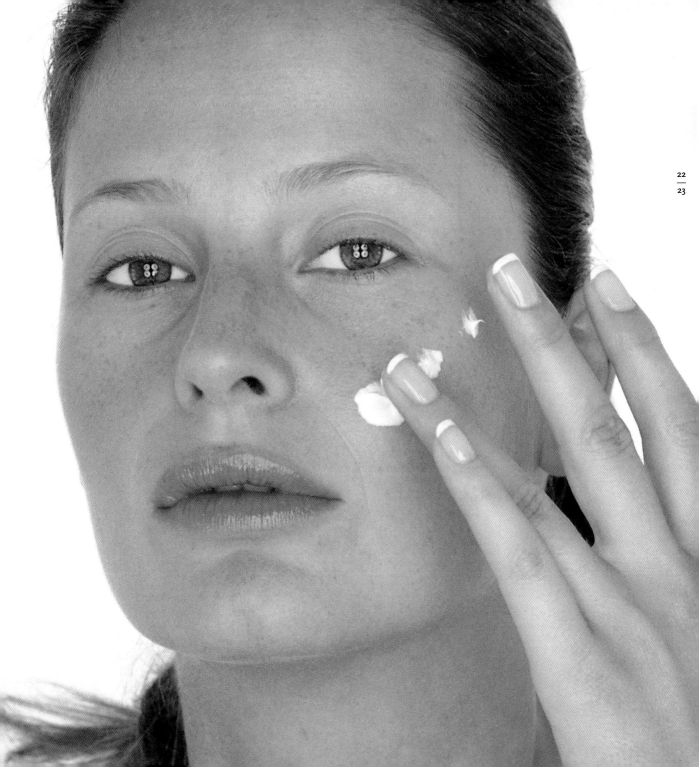

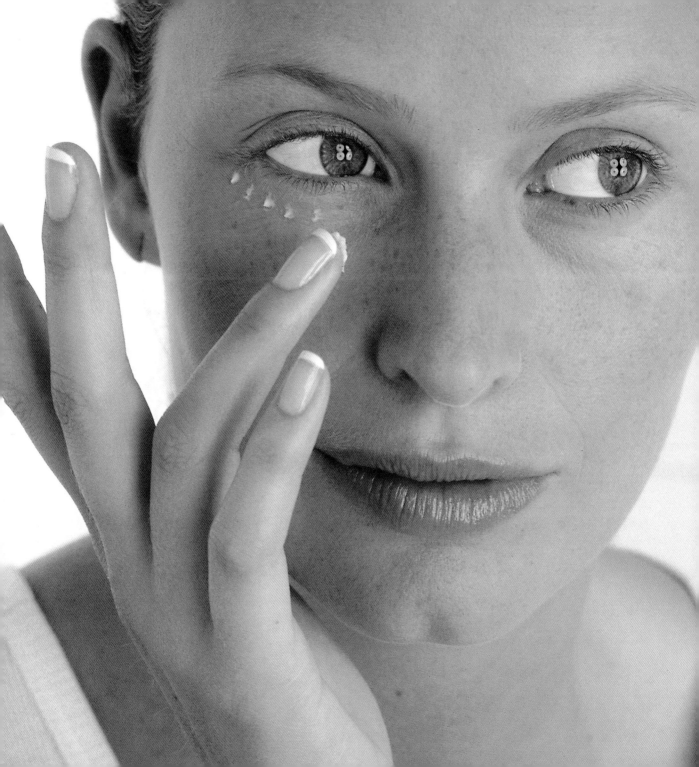

EYE CREAMS

The skin around the eyes is extremely delicate. It has no pores and thus cannot stay supple on its own. When choosing your eye cream you must again be objective about what your eyes really need. Are your eyes puffy? Do you have dark circles? These are two completely different problems. If your eyes retain water then you need a gel-based eye cream that contains a topical diuretic. Use this at night because gels are a little sticky and applying makeup over them can get gloppy. If you have dark circles, you can use a cream-based eye cream and fix the circles with concealer later. I have two eye creams. One for night and another, lighter version for day. I pat this underneath my eyes, being careful not to pull the delicate skin around them.

ALPHA-HYDROXY ACIDS

There are a number of new products on the market that contain fruit acids. These alpha-hydroxy acids exfoliate your skin by using the vitamins A or C from fruit to remove dead skin cells. Over-the-counter alpha-hydroxy products are never as strong as prescription products, so irritation should be minimal. But if you have very sensitive skin, consult a trusted dermatologist before using one. Keep in mind that you are accelerating the exfoliating process, so a certain amount of redness is normal after using them. You should avoid exposure to the sun while using these products, as the newly exposed skin is very sensitive—and sun damage is probably the reason why you'd need to start using the products in the first place!

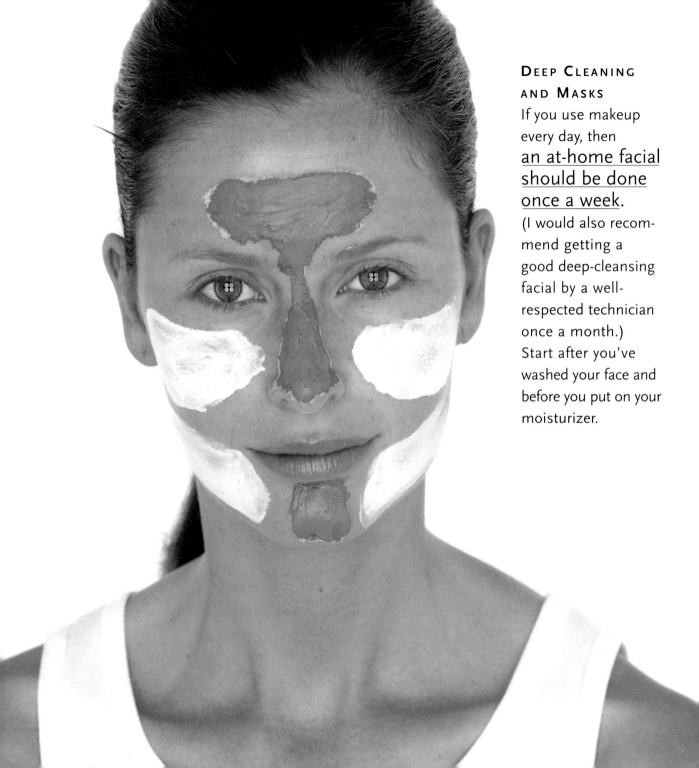

DEEP CLEANING AND MASKS

If you use makeup every day, then **an at-home facial should be done once a week.** (I would also recommend getting a good deep-cleansing facial by a well-respected technician once a month.) Start after you've washed your face and before you put on your moisturizer.

Allow your pores to open naturally by taking a nice, warm shower or placing a warm, moist washcloth over your face for at least 10 minutes. Don't steam your face. You could scald the skin.

While your face is still damp, use an exfoliating mask. Remember that if you use alpha-hydroxy products, Retin-A, or Vitamin C, another exfoliating mask might be too strong for your skin. You should skip this step and go directly to step 3, the deep-cleansing mask. If you don't use exfoliating creams, you can try either an almond mask that has some raw almond in it or a peeling mask that sinks into the skin before being peeled or rubbed off. Just make sure that you peel small sections at a time and that you use both hands when removing the mask: one keeping your skin taut and the other rubbing lightly in small circles. There are dozens of these masks; I recommend you find one that contains the purest ingredients possible.

After you exfoliate you should deep clean the oily parts of your skin with a mud, algae, or charcoal mask and the dry parts with a moisturizing and hydrating mask.

Rinse first with warm water and then cool water.

Dab some drying mask on the parts of your face that are extremely oily or places where you have existing pimples. Then apply a calming mask all over your face. A good calming mask will contain chamomile, cucumber, or comfrey—natural products that will make your skin silky and reduce the redness that may have appeared because of the intensity of this facial. Masks and topical creams are very important for the face, as they will help to keep your pores clean. Dirt in a pore will stretch it out, and as you age, the skin around the pores won't spring back like it did in your youth.

Notice that I never recommend that you pick or squeeze any whiteheads or blackheads. If your pores are opened from the shower and then you use the exfoliating mask you should naturally get rid of some of those pimples. If not, the addition of drying lotions should do the trick. If you feel that your whiteheads, blackheads, and pimples are not budging and you must squeeze, my advice is that you go to a professional facialist and invest in that process. I cannot stress enough the importance of letting a professional do that kind of extraction.

Dirt in
your pores
will stretch
them out
over time.
As you
age, the
skin around
them won't
spring
back as it
did in your
youth.

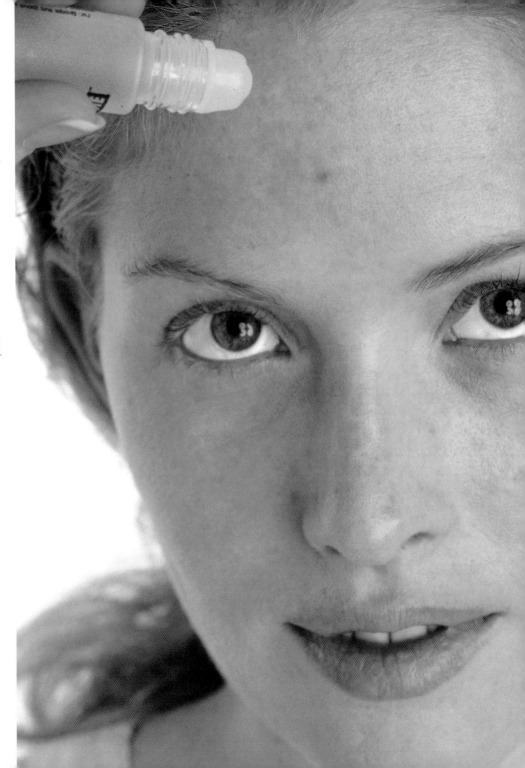

solutions to your common skin problems

UNEVEN PIGMENT

Uneven pigment has many causes. Years of sun exposure and the natural aging process will leave some people with skin discoloration. Some birth-control pills can cause hyperpigmentation. Alpha-hydroxy products work on minor discoloration but for a more severe case you can use a skin lightening lotion. There are many over-the-counter forms of skin-bleaching creams that have a minute amount of hydroquinone or kojic acid, which actually stops the production of melanin, rather than bleaching the skin as chlorine would bleach a shirt. You must be careful when using bleaching creams in conjunction with other hyper-exfoliating creams because combining the two can make your skin extra-sensitive to the sun. When this happens you can end up with greater discoloration than you

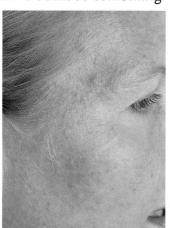

started with. Start with a very mild skin bleaching cream; if it doesn't work, gradually switch to stronger products. Bleaching creams can cause side effects, so if it's a mild case, use concealers to fix the problem.

TEENAGE SKIN

Teenage skin is often oily and can be particularly prone to breakouts because of all the hormones rumbling around the area. So it is especially important for teenagers to keep their faces and hands clean all the time. That means you can really never touch your face. And as I said before, if you pick your pimples now, you will have scars to hide later on in life. You should also wash your face several times during the day. An oil-free moisturizer is a must, and I would also recommend using an alcohol-free toner after washing and throughout the day. It's easy to keep a small travel-size bottle of toner with cotton balls handy to keep your skin clean.

BLEMISHES

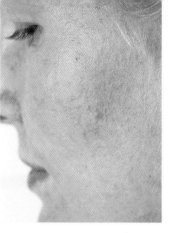

When a blemish appears on my skin, I apply a tiny amount of tea tree oil directly to it with a cotton swab. In its purest form, tea tree oil is very strong, so you have to be careful not to use too much or it can be very drying. If you are going to wear makeup, simply put the tea tree oil or a drying spot lotion under your primer, taking care to dab it only where the pimple is. This precise application will avoid the circle that a finger-tip application will leave.

CYSTIC ACNE

People with cystic acne are usually fair skinned, of Northern European origin. Their strong, thick skin has a lot of collagen that prevents pimples from coming up to the top layer of skin, so they fester underneath and become worse. Scrubbing the face won't break through that layer, so topical treatments such as alpha-hydroxy acids are the only source of relief. The fruit acid exfoliates the skin from underneath the derma (top layer of skin), so it helps bring up the underlying acne. With this type of skin I would always seek guidance from a dermatologist, who can also advise you on the different peels available for skin resurfacing if you have scars. The good news is that this type of skin heals well and quickly.

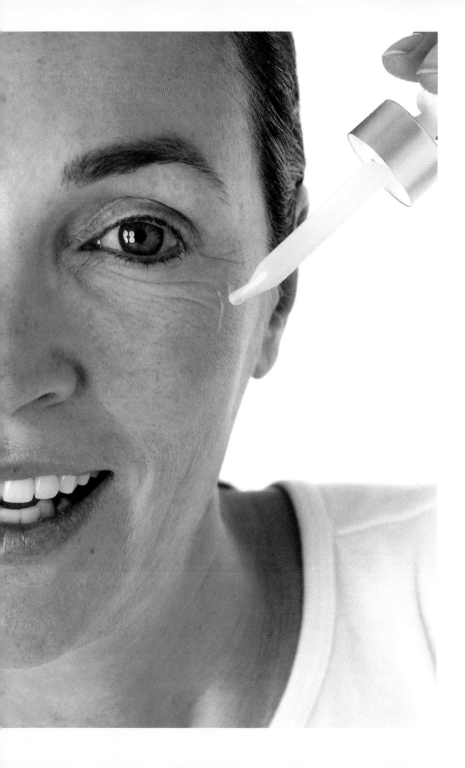

AGING SKIN

Wrinkles are the early signs of age. When you first start seeing them on your face, begin to investigate mild over-the-counter alpha-hydroxy acids. These products will help exfoliate your skin, smoothing out some of the fine lines and evening out some pigment differences. To treat more advanced signs of age, refer to the Dr. Griffin box on the following pages for information on other options and treatments.

*I have a wonderful der-
matologist, Dr. Edmond
Griffin, who has been
treating my different skin
problems for many years.
He's a wealth of infor-
mation and I asked him
to explain what all the
new products can do for
you and what treatments
are available. Throughout
the book I will refer to
Dr. Griffin for different
questions that you might
have concerning skin,
aging, products, cosmetic
surgery, and other issues
for which a professional
opinion will be helpful.*

Which treatments will help diminish the early signs of aging?

Topical fruit-acid peels or micro-sponge salicylic acid peels can be used to remove the dead layer of skin. These peels have the advantage of safety and lack of downtime as compared to the trichloroacetic acid peels. The regular use of one of the retinoic acid creams (Retin-A, Renova) and glycolic acid creams completes your initial program of treatment and prevention of those early signs of aging. Botox is now coming to the aid of the younger person with frown lines and early crow's feet due to frowning or squinting. Collagen injections (both the human-tissue matrix type and calf collagen) can also be used for those earliest wrinkles.

What are chemical peels?

Chemical peels have been used to rejuvenate the skin since the time of the Egyptians. Chemical peels are commonly divided into superficial, medium, and deep peels. The results that can be expected with the superficial peel include improvement in skin texture and color and some fine-line softening. A medium-depth peel improves blotchy pigmentation, sun damage, fine wrinkles, and some acne scars, and has effect on deeper wrinkling. Deep chemical peels, such as the phenol peels, are not used as frequently since the development of laser skin resurfacing, which is now the treatment of choice for deep wrinkling, extensive sun damage, and acne scarring.

Some people, as they age, notice increased blood vessels, a redder nose, and the return of acne, especially on their noses and cheeks. What can be done?

The symptoms suggest a condition known as rosacea. Laser treatments can eradicate the blood vessels easily, with no scarring and minimal downtime. Antibiotics are usually necessary to eliminate the acne pimples.

There are so many peels now, how will a woman know what she needs?
The appropriate peel depends upon a woman's age, the extent of sun damage to her skin, and the amount of downtime she has available. The younger person may prefer to use weaker acids more often rather than moderate acids with a longer downtime and more risks. An older patient with severe sun damage has to consider more downtime, more risks, and more costs to reverse the damage by using the strongest acids (or dermabrasions, or laser resurfacing).

Laser for wrinkles means a quick treatment requiring little anesthetic and fast recovery?
Wrong! This is a common misconception about laser resurfacing. Because wrinkles and photodamage extend deeply into the layers of skin, the laser must destroy the skin and the body must restore it back to a healthy and more youthful look with increased collagen and elastic fibers. This depth requires usually both sedation and anesthesia.

What can a woman do if she can't take time off work but wants to improve her skin?
Besides sunscreens, glycolic acid creams, and retinoic acid cream one can consider the lunchtime peels with glycolic acid or even the combination formula known as Jessner's solution or the microsponge salicylic acid peels. Most recently the rage has been the microdermabrasion with aluminum crystals.

Can you mix techniques in facial rejuvenation?
Not only can you mix, you may only get ideal results if you do so. In areas where the surgeon can be less aggressive he or she may choose medium-strength chemical peeling and use both laser resurfacing and dermabrasion on the deep resistant wrinkles of the upper lip.

don't be
embarrassed,
the truth is
that everyone
has
hair follicles
on their face

facial hair

People get embarrassed about facial hair, but the truth is that everyone has hair follicles on their face. I'm always very open when discussing my own facial hair, so I don't mind telling other women that the excess hair over their lip or around their eyebrows has got to go. There are many ways to deal with unwanted hair. I have fine blond peach fuzz on most of my face. Around my upper lip there are some darker hairs. I have very sensitive skin and I break out if I wax my top lip, so when

I'm shooting a beauty job, I snip the darker hairs with small scissors. My mother has her top lip and eyebrows waxed every eight weeks. She has no reaction, and because her eyesight is not great, plucking her own eyebrows could spell disaster.

BLEACHING

If you have darker peach fuzz all over your face or a low line of hair on your forehead you may want to investigate over-the-counter bleaching products. I have used these products on many clients to lighten hair around the forehead line or even the brow line if the hair continues up over the forehead. I don't usually recommend using a bleaching cream for longer facial hair because the hair will still be long. You may not notice it, but others will.

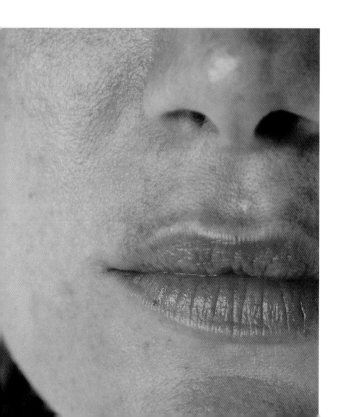

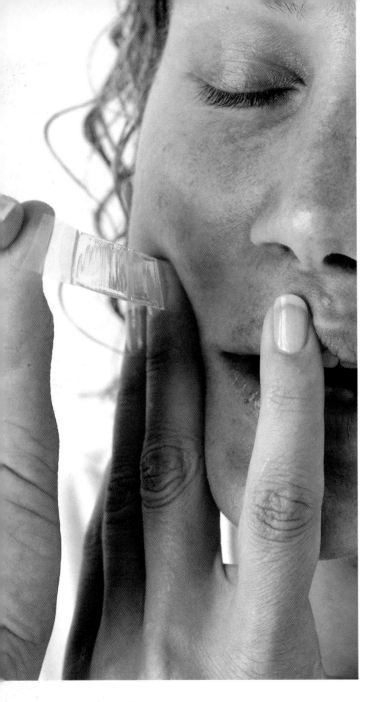

WAXING

In my opinion, waxing is the easiest way to get rid of unwanted hair. But the skin on the face is very delicate and a reaction to wax could cause scarring and skin discoloration, so you may not want to wax your face yourself the first time. Professional waxing has become quite popular, so it's available almost everywhere and the prices have come down. But if you want to do your waxing at home, there are some great cold waxes on the market now.

One of the worst old wives' tales is that if you wax or snip the hairs on your face they will grow back darker and thicker. Your hair type is determined by genetics. The reason it seems darker after regrowing is because the old hair was lightened by the sun over time. The reason it seems thicker is because you see it grow back all at once. Don't worry. If you want a smooth appearance on your face you have to keep this process up—usually every eight weeks. Or you can invest in other, more permanent hair removal processes.

ELECTROLYSIS

Electrolysis is the process of killing the individual hair follicles with an electric shock. It is a good alternative to waxing because it's more permanent, although you will need to have the process done several times for it to work. It's expensive, though, and the prices never seem to go down. It can also be time-consuming, since you can only do small patches at a time.

LASER TREATMENT

This process is similar to electrolysis. Instead of an electric shock killing the follicle, a laser light is used. Some people swear by it and others say that it really only lasts six months. It's also very expensive. Like electrolysis, it takes some time for complete results, as only a small area can be treated each session. Go to a laser-treatment professional who comes highly recommended and whose results you've seen and liked.

TWEEZING

The best technique for maintenance of hair removal in small areas is tweezing. Just be sure you clean the area first with alcohol and cotton balls. Refer to "Elementary Eyebrows" in chapter 2.

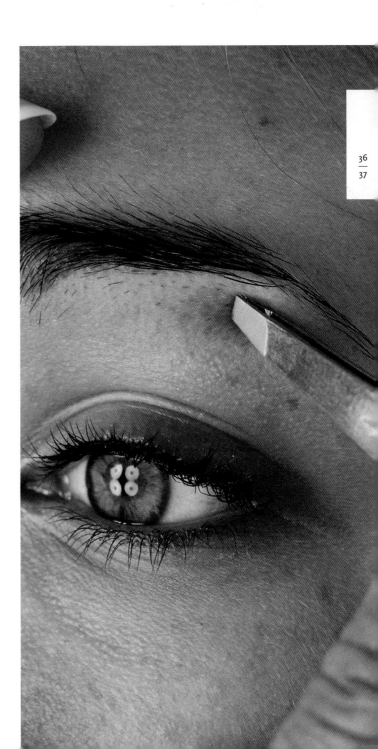

the sun

We are inundated with information about the effects of the sun on skin. The bottom line is that the sun is the second most harmful factor to your skin after smoking. Exposure to the sun serves to drain the collagen and hydration out of your skin. If you are going to take care of your skin by cleaning and moisturizing correctly, why undo it by not protecting against the sun?

I'll be the first one to say that I look better when my skin is a little "sun-kissed." But I watch very carefully how much sun I get. I use a sunscreen every day. I do not recommend sunbathing but I will say that when I'm at the beach I use the highest SPF I can get, one that contains titanium dioxide. As there is no such thing as a safe tan, I try to be conscientious while I still have fun outdoors. Take advantage of one of the many sunless tanners on the market, which can give you as healthy-looking a tan as you see in the swimsuit catalogs.

SUNLESS TANNING

There are some great tanners on the market today, and they don't use the old carrot dye anymore so you won't look like an orange.

The formulas are also much better smelling now. You should experiment to find the right one for you. I use a different tanner for my body and my face, because the skin on my face is very sensitive and oily. I usually keep my face a little lighter and use bronzing makeup to enhance my sun-kissed glow. Jillian also likes the sun-kissed look but wants to protect her skin.

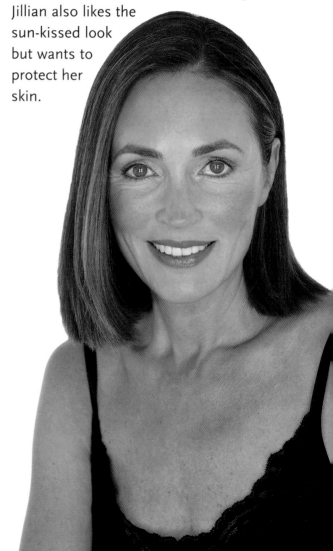

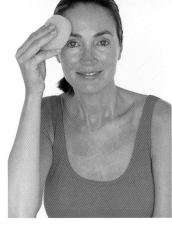

The first step is to prepare the skin. Just as our faces have oil spots and dry spots, so do our bodies. There are places where the tanner is absorbed faster and deeper. While in the shower take a loofah or other exfoliant and scrub your skin in little circles, paying particular attention to your knees and elbows, which get very dry from all the bending they do.

Dry off and sit down on a dark towel. Use petroleum jelly on the bottoms of your feet to protect them from the tanning cream. Then, using circular motions, spread the cream or oil with your fingers evenly over your

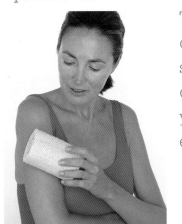

body one section at a time, starting with your feet. As you move up your body, use a mirror to check that you haven't missed any spots and that the application is even. Stand up when it's time to do your back and shoulders.

If you need it all over you should have another person apply it to your back. If you do it yourself, use a small amount and apply it with your fingertips to the middle of your back.

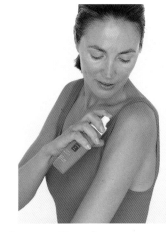

Wash your hands immediately. They will probably still get a little stained but it will come off. You can use surgical gloves to apply the tanner, if you have them handy.

It takes about an hour to see the results of your effort. If you wish to be darker still you can reapply the next day.

Which sunscreen is best?

You need a "broad-spectrum" blocker that provides coverage for both UVA and UVB. At present, there is no established way to judge a sunscreen's ability to protect against UVA. The SPF measures only its protection against the UVB ultraviolet light. Even the highest SPF sunscreens do not provide 100 percent protection. Always read the labels. The blocker Avobenzone Parsol 1789, recently approved by the FDA, is touted as the best UVA blocker. Other blockers of UVA light are the micronized titanium and zinc formulas.

When is a tan healthy?

The tanning industry would have you believe that a tan is healthy. In truth a tan is proof that damage has occurred and the body has produced melanin for protection. If you do not tan easily, you will receive the most ultraviolet damage. If you burn easily, you will wrinkle easily.

Can't I just get a little color before applying my sunscreen?

Sun damage starts in minutes and its effects last a lifetime. There is no grace period before you cover up. In time, sags and wrinkles appear after these unprotected brief exposures. You need to protect the main structural proteins of the skin: elastin and collagen. Apply sunscreen at least thirty minutes before intense exposure, and don't expose your skin during the peak UVA and UVB times of the day, from 11:00 A.M. to 3:00 P.M. No sunscreens offer full protection, so if you must be in the sun, use protective clothing and hats.

Who is most at risk for developing skin cancer?

People who are particularly at risk are those who have had three or more blistering sunburns before the age of twenty, have multiple large moles on the body, have fair complexions, have developed scaly red spots on sun-exposed areas, and have been weekend sun worshippers.

If my skin damage is developing from sun exposure that happened years ago, why worry now?

Evidence is clear that current sun damage aggravates former damage and speeds its progression to skin cancer.

Are tanning beds safer than natural sun?

No. The latest information shows that it is UVA, the wavelength given off by the sunbeds, that is particularly responsible for skin cancers and sun-damaged skin.

On cloudy days do I need a sunscreen?

Yes. Eighty percent of the sun's ultraviolet rays, especially UVA, can penetrate clouds.

What other factors break down the skin and produce damage?

Smoke, pollutants, pesticides, herbicides, and extreme heat and cold all produce damaging, reactive, oxygen-based molecules, better known as free radicals. Try to avoid these harmful environmental conditions.

What are the signs of skin cancer?

The rule is simple: any changing mole, any new mole, any sore that does not heal, any new growth that is red, itchy, and bleeding. A skilled dermatologist can easily differentiate between the normal and the dangerous, but you must also perform self-exams, looking carefully and regularly for changes in moles or new marks on your skin. Ask your partner or spouse to look you over now and then, especially in areas that are difficult to see yourself. The best time for this inspection is at bath time under bright lights. If you find anything suspicious, call your dermatologist.

your makeup

Creating a beautiful face can be so much fun. With makeup, you can completely change your look. You can be Sophia Loren or Cleopatra. You can use makeup to de-emphasize the features you don't like and enhance those you do like. The important thing to remember is that <u>you want your *features* to stand out, not your makeup.</u> When looking in catalogs, you will hardly ever be able to see a model's makeup. They all have it on, but it's not the makeup that's supposed to look beautiful, it's the model. That's the look we'll aim for.

When a model is on a job, her makeup artist will have to deal with a myriad of different skin conditions, from pimples to drastic pigmentation variations. All of this can be fixed with the magic of makeup. In this chapter, I'll offer solutions to these problems.

Looking in the mirror is the first step. Decide what you like and what you'd like to change. Honestly evaluate your strong and weak points. I will show you how to use makeup to enhance the strong features and de-emphasize the weak ones. You'll learn how to do your own basic face, the five-minute face for the woman on the go, and makeup for such special events as your wedding day.

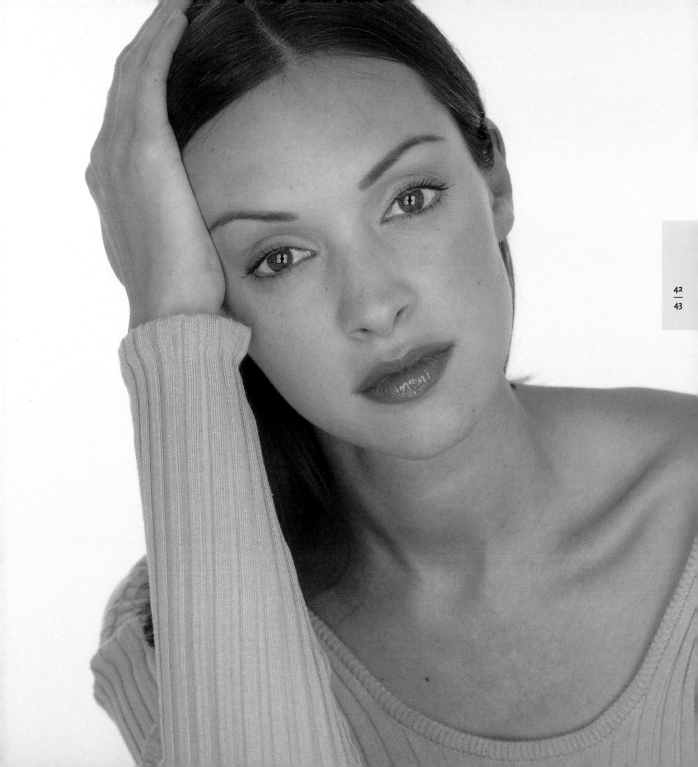

your basic face

You can follow these easy steps for your everyday face or use this as a starting place for more advanced or different looks. We will refer back to the basic face often in this chapter.

MOISTURIZER

It's important to start with clean, moisturized skin. Use a light moisturizer with a sunscreen already in it; oil-free moisturizers are a good choice. If you have problematic or volatile skin, you should be specific about where you apply the moisturizer, applying where your skin is dry and avoiding blemishes. You can dilute the moisturizer with a little water, or apply your moisturizer while your skin is still damp from washing. This not only seals in the moisture, but also helps oily, problem skin absorb the cream without feeling too heavy.

PRIMER

I begin my makeup application with a primer. A primer is a non-oily cream that seals the moisturizer in your skin, forming a barrier between the moisturizer and the makeup, creating a smooth surface for the foundation or concealer. One that has botanicals in it can also alleviate puffiness and shrink the pores slightly. Primer also helps your makeup last all day without fading. If you need to clean up or reshape your eyebrows, now is the time. Refer to "Elementary Eyebrows" on page 56.

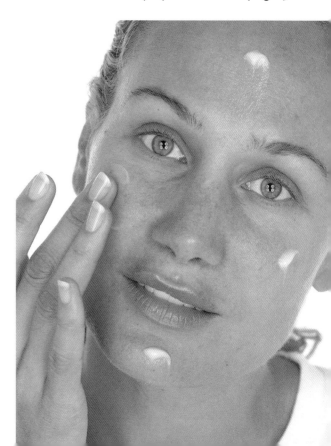

FOUNDATION

I'm not a huge fan of foundation. It is very hard to find the perfect color for an entire face and this usually means that you end up looking like you're wearing a mask. Plus, the more products you put over your acne, the more acne you may produce. It is a wise idea to fix the acne and use only minimal coverage. Heavy products will also sink into fine lines and wrinkles and make them more noticeable. I did not use foundation on any of the makeovers I did in this book—not because the women we selected had perfect skin, but because I believe that most women don't need coverage all over. If you are used to using foundation you can read on; if you want to use concealer only where you truly need it, skip to the concealer section.

Foundation is used to give your skin a uniform tone, so finding a foundation that truly matches your skin is critical. It is best to use natural sunlight to test the color. Don't test the color on your hand, because your hands usually get more sun than your face, so it will never be quite the right match. Instead, use the side of your jawbone. Your foundation should be applied sheerly. Most people only have certain areas on their face that need to be concealed, so don't cover your skin excessively where you don't need it. It looks unnatural. Think about house paint; foundation should look more like sheer stain than thick latex. You should see your skin through it.

Applying from the center of your nose and working outward, deposit more foundation where you need it most. Avoid applying foundation around the eye—coverage with the concealer will be plenty. And keep in mind that your face does not end at your jaw line; with your sponge, apply foundation under your chin and down your neck. If you apply it correctly, with no distinct lines, it will not be obvious.

If you have very bad acne and a sheer foundation doesn't seem to cover enough, you can try a dual foundation. This is a foundation designed to be applied wet or dry. If you apply it wet, it will cover like a pancake makeup; dry, it is like a thick pressed powder. Dual foundation should be used only for drastic pigmentation problems or rosacea that cannot be covered with a good concealer. The foundation will, obviously, show up; long-term solutions for this type of problem skin are discussed in chapter one.

CONCEALER

Many women don't want to use concealers because they hate the covered-up, overly made-up look. But this can be avoided by using a pigment-rich concealer. "Pigment-rich" means that all the weight in the concealer is in the color. Concealer is designed to cover flaws with a concentrated amount of pigment. Some areas of the facial skin are thinner than others. Our skin is thinnest under the eye, and sometimes the veins will show through. Instead of applying a heavy coat of foundation you can use a concealer and just concentrate on specific areas. You don't want it to be soft or creamy, because that means there are moisturizers, humectants, talc, perfume, or oils in it. Any of these will make it slip and slide on your blemishes and will also add oil to an already irritated spot. Also, <u>your body temperature is 98.6 degrees Fahrenheit; the combination of the heat and gravity can make the concealer slide right down your face</u>. The perfect concealer is thick and dry to the touch. It is best to apply it with a thin, flat, synthetic brush, as the oil in your fingers will change the color of the concealer. You should warm it up a little by dabbing it with a brush. If you're using a high-pigment concealer, you won't

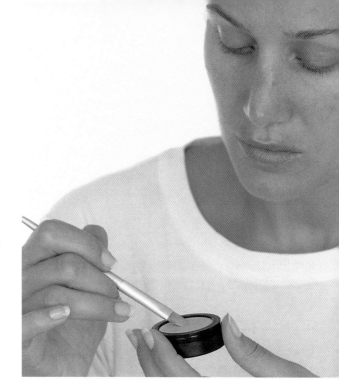

need to use much to achieve good coverage.

Finding a concealer that is the correct color can be difficult. The best way is to find a two-toned concealer set: one concealer that closely matches your skin tone and another that is a light yellow tone to cancel out the red or blue tones that you'll be covering up. Practice makes perfect in this area and you'll quickly be able to determine the color and tone that work for you. Keep in mind that a rose-based color cancels gray tones in the skin, and a yellow base cancels blue and red.

1 Holding the brush like a painter would, brush on the concealer in light, sweeping, flat 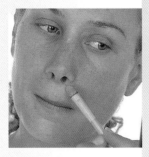 strokes, lifting after you've covered each spot. Try to use strokes so light that there will be no need to pat down the concealer to blend.

2 After you've covered all blemishes, spider veins, brown spots, and so on, move on to the area under the eye. This is the most delicate tissue on your face, the first place to lose collagen and oil (which is why we get wrinkles here first). Add a small dab of non–gel-based eye cream to the concealer and blend with the brush. Applying the mixture and using little feather strokes under the inside corner of the eye, you'll see the redness slowly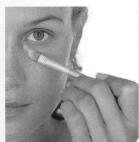

disappear. Don't overdo it! Only cover the red or blue part, being careful not to apply the concealer too far out. Women have a tendency to sweep concealer all the way out to the edge of the eye, but the skin is usually not red or dark there, so all this does is add pigment to the wrinkles on the outside of the eye, accentuating them further.

3 Finally, take a little concealer and pat your ring finger on it. Transfer it from your ring finger to the closed lid. Pat lightly. This is a good way to lighten up the lid and not pull the skin. It's also great for women who wear contacts because a brush could dislodge the lens. Once your concealer is applied, you're ready to move onto powder.

POWDER

Powder sets your foundation and/or concealer; the dryness picks up any moisture and oil that is on your skin, leaving a smooth surface for adding other powder-based color. It is

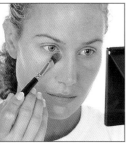

important to use clear translucent powder because it is the lightest available. Remember that when you add any pigment, you add weight; this only results in an overly made-up look and actually brings out fine lines and wrinkles.

There is some debate over the use of clear translucent powder versus yellow powder. I only use powder with pigment where my face is relatively flat—cheeks, forehead, jawbone. Everywhere else the face has natural creases —under the eye, sides of the nose, and around the mouth—and adding a pigmented powder will only deepen the shadows caused by the creases. I use only clear translucent powder in these areas. Remember that you're already using foundation and concealer with a yellow base. Using powder with a yellow base could make you look sallow. If you need yellow powder, the concealer isn't working.

Dip a synthetic brush (one that is never used with colored powder) lightly into the powder. Tap the excess off the brush or puff and lightly sweep the powder over the area. Remember, powder is used to set your makeup, not cover your skin like a blanket. If the clear translucent powder looks white once applied, you're using too much.

There is also a debate on whether loose or pressed powder is best. Loose powder has the least amount of fillers. In order to "press" a powder, a binder, such as oil or wax, has to be added so that the powder stays firm. I prefer loose powder, so that I know I'll be adding as little to my skin as possible. If you simply must carry a pressed powder, use it only where your face is flat (where you'd put colored powder) and also be very careful if you have sensitive, acne-prone skin, as the added fillers may clog your pores and give you more acne to cover up.

Take the brush and lightly set the places where you used concealer. Don't worry about the entire face (when adding blush and contouring, you'll be powdering the rest of the face plenty). I don't like the over-powdered look. I prefer to look a little dewy. If you do like to look completely powdered, then take a puff and pat the entire face lightly with translucent powder.

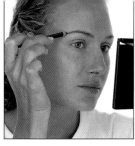

FILLING IN YOUR EYEBROWS

The shape of your eyebrow is only one part of what eyebrows can do for you. The color is also very important. You have to make sure you complement your face with the color of your eyebrows, and this is best done by choosing a color that is similar to your hair. If you have ash in your base hair color, pick an eyebrow color that is also ash based, even if you want to slightly lighten your brows. Follow the same rule if you have red tones in your hair, even if you are darkening your brows.

INVISIBLE EYELINER AND YOUR BASIC SHADOW

1 With a sharpened eye pencil draw a line as close to the root of your upper lashes as possible. Take your ring finger and hold the eyelid so you can jiggle the pencil tip into your roots. This creates a darker and thicker lash root line, without showing the eyeliner itself. You want to keep the pencil inside the lashes so that there is no color on top of the lid (liner on the lids will make your eye look smaller).

2 With a flat, square-tipped synthetic brush use either a wet liner or create a wet liner with a little water on your dry shadow. Make it as dense as possible and jiggle the brush into your lashes just as you did with the pencil. This will further intensify your line.

3 Choose a shadow color that's only a few shades darker than your own skin color and apply with a soft-tip, natural-hair brush. With your eyes open, follow slightly above your natural crease. This opens up the eye and gives it subtle shading.

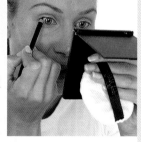

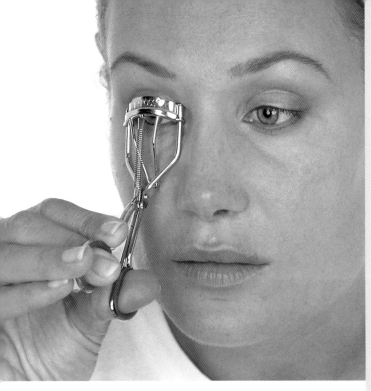

1 While looking in the mirror, guide the opened curler as close to the base of your lashes as possible, being careful not to get any skin inside.

2 Keeping your hand very still, close the curler for a few seconds.

3 Release and pull the curler out until only a third of your lash tip is still in the curler.

4 Close the curler again. This prevents the crimped, one-bend look.

EYELASH CURLING

I can't tell you what an amazing difference this simple contraption makes. Most models will forego almost any other part of the makeup if they can have curled lashes! An eyelash curler bends lashes that naturally point downward. This opens up the eye and slightly separates the lashes.

When shopping for an eyelash curler, look for one with a soft, sponge rubber rim, so no metal will touch your lashes. It should fit the eye socket without pulling the outside lashes.

MASCARA

Choosing mascara is difficult. Models are experts at this because we usually bring our own to every shoot. For sanitary reasons, you should never share a mascara wand. The infections that can be passed on are potentially very dangerous.

Understanding what you really need is important, so take a good look at your lashes. Are they light colored? Most women just need a good, dark, highly pigmented mascara to cover light lashes. If you have very fair skin and don't wear much makeup, you should use a brown mascara.

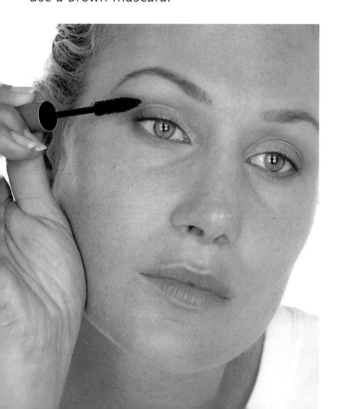

I recommend a non-filler, high-pigmented mascara. Before applying, be sure to wipe a little of the color off the wand first. Start at the root of your lash, gently jiggling the wand so it coats as close to the root as possible. Between this and the pencil liner that you just applied to the lash line, you should have no nude space under the lashes. You want to create a beautifully framed eye, without the weight. If your lashes are sparse and short, you will need mascara that will build your lashes and make them look longer.

Be aware that mascara made with fillers and polyester look great when you apply them, but an hour later, after the water and wax have dried, the polyester and filler that made your lashes look longer can flake off and make dark circles under your eyes. The last thing you want is spider lashes.

When you're finished with your makeup you can apply false eyelashes, even if you don't use thick liner (see page 81). This is just to open up close-set eyes (like mine).

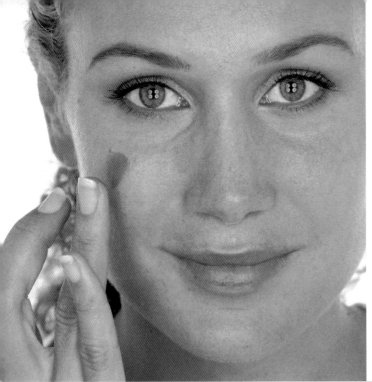

you really do blush. Your blush should harmonize with your skin, not compete with it.

If you just love your powder blush, take a natural-hair blush brush and lay it flat on the color. Tap off a little and then lay it flat on the apple of your cheek and gently pull down. Don't smash it into your cheek, but lightly stroke with downward pulls of the brush directly on the apple. Any contouring that you wish to do should be done with a powder closer to your foundation color.

For acne-prone skin I recommend a gel-based blush. Usually these are water-based and much less occlusive (pore clogging).

Blush

Blush should not be applied to your cheek-bones or your chin, but to the apple of your cheeks—where you blush. If you need a guide, simply smile.

I recommend using a cream or liquid blush, to be applied after your concealer and before your powder. It will give you a youthful, dewy look. Sometimes too much powder on the face begins to look like crepe paper. When choosing a color, determine if your complexion is yellow or rosy. Select a color that is close to the color your skin becomes when

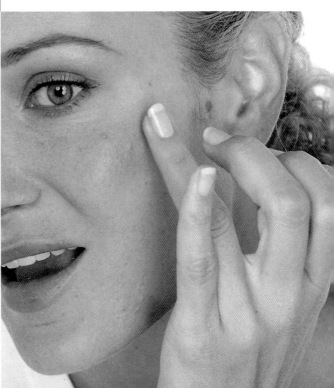

What common irritants found in cosmetics could cause or aggravate acne?
Comedogenicity is the term used if an ingredient produces blackheads, whiteheads, or acne. One should purchase ingredients tested for comedogenicity especially if acne prone. Keep in mind that oil-free products do not necessarily mean non-comedogenic.

Why would someone develop a rash after using a hypoallergenic cosmetic?
Skin rashes usually represent an irritant reaction and not an allergic one. The main cosmetics causing irritant contact dermatitis include soaps, eye shadow, mascara, shampoos, permanent hair wave products, and certain moisturizers. The most common cosmetic allergens are fragrances, preservatives, and hair dyes. Patch testing can be performed to look for any possible allergens.

What is the best treatment for dark circles under the eyes?
New information shows that a vitamin K cream in combination with retinoic acid may improve these circles. If you have genetic dark circles, this is most likely from extra pigment within the skin, and bleaching creams may reduce the extra pigment. More advanced treatments include strong acid peels, laser resurfacing with the CO_2 laser, or pigment reduction with the Q-switched ruby laser. Finally, because some of the discoloration originates from the blood vessel surrounding the fat pads of the eyelids, a lower eyelid surgery (biepharoplasty) will reduce this type of discoloration.

How would I choose the right treatment for my eyelids?
Unless your discoloration comes and goes with allergies, fatigue level, and alcohol consumption (in which case eyelid surgery is an option), dark circles are probably due to melanin in the skin and not blood vessels under your skin. These will be helped best by bleaching and lightening techniques.

ask
Dr. Griffin

?

LIPSTICK

There are two ridges to your lips: the natural and the color ridge. Usually the color ridge is slightly smaller than the natural ridge. If you look in the mirror at a three-quarter profile, you'll see the natural ridge. It's the raised part that defines your lips. Most women line their lips using the color ridge only as a guide. But when you do this, you automatically make your lips look smaller. The color ridge also recedes as we age, making it appear as if our lips are shrinking, when it's really just the color ridge fading. When you line your lip, look for the natural ridge.

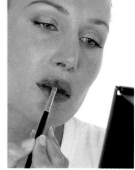

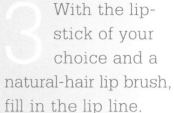

1   Once you've concealed both your color and natural ridges, use a little powder to set the concealer.

2   Carefully line the ridge with a lip pencil (I prefer a nude, almost lip-colored pencil). Then fill in the rest of your lip with the liner.

3   With the lipstick of your choice and a natural-hair lip brush, fill in the lip line. This brush should be a little stiff, but not so stiff that it scratches you. When you are in a hurry, you can forgo the brush, but while you're getting used to defining your lip ridge by the natural line, I suggest you use it.

4   Blot your lip with a single sheet of tissue. After blotting, you can sweep a little powder over the lip and add another coat. I'm not crazy about the stay-on lip colors because they are silicone-based and tend to dry out your lips. The blotting technique with re-application usually stains the lip, so you won't have to reapply as often.

5   Just add some sheer lip gloss to polish the look and off you go!

Once you have finished applying your makeup, take a look at yourself in a natural light, or whatever light is closest to the light you spend most of your day in. Judge how much makeup you really need. Remember that your skin is an organ that has to breathe. If you have too much makeup on your face, it will either push it off or absorb it. Try to keep this in mind when selecting foundations and concealers. Go for more pigment and less filler (emollients, perfume, oil, talc). Use as little as possible to get the coverage you need.

Keep an open mind when experimenting with makeup. The industry has become much more skin-friendly, as well as more receptive to how women want their faces to look. I'm always reading magazines and watching for new products. When you see something in a magazine that you like, give it a try. It might just become part of the "new you."

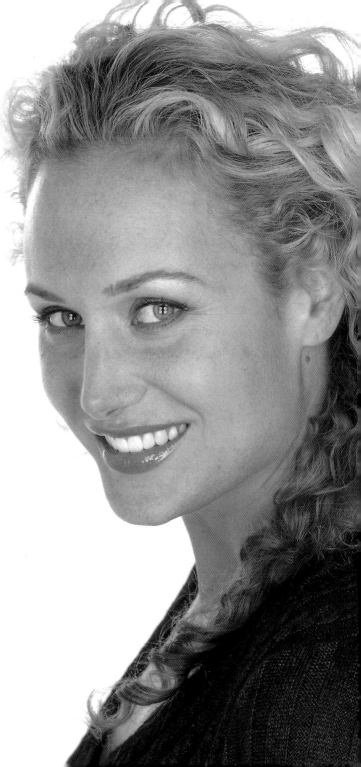

Elementary Eyebrows

Eyebrows frame the top of your face, just as your jawbone frames the bottom. Shaping your eyebrows is a process that can be done two ways: a professional can wax, thread, or use electrolysis to shape your brows, or you can shape them yourself with tweezers. I do not recommend waxing them yourself—wax is hot and applying it close to the eye is risky. Shaping them with tweezers is easy.

I prefer a slant-edged tweezer with a slightly textured, rough point that grasps the hair easily. You shouldn't have to grab the hair too tightly for the tweezers to work.

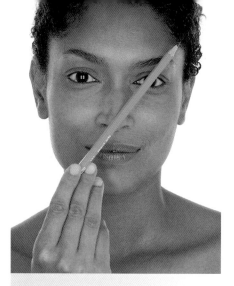

hot tip

WHEN EXTENDING THE BROW TOWARD YOUR TEMPLE, LIFT THE SKIN ABOVE THE BROW WITH YOUR FINGER. INSTEAD OF DRAWING THE LINE DOWNWARD, DRAW IT STRAIGHT OUT AND VERY SLIGHTLY DOWN. WHEN YOU RELEASE YOUR FINGER, THE BROW SHOULD CURVE DOWN GENTLY.

1 Looking straight into a mirror, take a pencil or long brush and hold it vertically in front of your face. Leaving the bottom of the pencil on the tip of your nose, turn the pencil to the right, like a clock hand sweeping the numbers from 12 o'clock to about 2 o'clock. As you look in the mirror, locate your iris, the colored part of your eyeball. Align the pencil tip with the iris; where it intersects your brow is where the highest part of your brow arch should be. Take a white pencil and mark this point at the top of your brow.

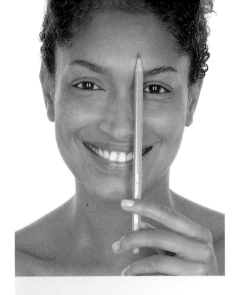

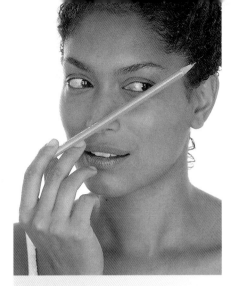

2 Align the pencil vertically with the innermost corner of your eye, where your tear duct is. Where the pencil intersects the eyebrow is where the brow should start. If your eyebrow starts much farther in than this, it will draw your eyes closer together, so if you have close-set eyes, mark this point to indicate where the brow should begin. Tweeze your brows up to that point. If your eyes are very wide apart you may want to balance the two points by using a pencil or some shadow and filling in each brow toward the nose.

3 Rest one end of the pencil on the tip of your nose, and the other on the outside corner of your eye. Where the pencil intersects the brow is where the brow should end. Most brows don't quite make it to this line. A brow pencil or some shadow can extend this line to balance a large jawbone and open up your eyes.

4 To make a very straight brow appear more arched, tweeze the top of the beginning of the brow so that it dips slightly lower than the arch over the iris. This will open up the eye.

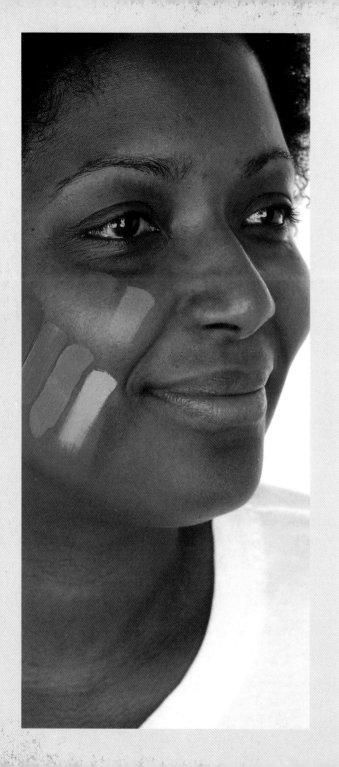

tips and solutions to common makeup problems

HOW TO CHOOSE THE RIGHT FOUNDATION/CONCEALER:

Finding the right foundation when you have different skin tones is a total drag. What may seem dark enough or the right tone in the bottle will look completely different on your skin. A foundation that looks yellow or golden on the shelf can look ashy on your skin. Try to find a department store or boutique where you can try the colors on your skin in natural light.

If a foundation is made correctly for darker skin, it should have a very high concentration of pigment. This will result in a very thick, rich consistency. With this in mind, know that you should apply it like you would a concealer: only where you really need it.

Marie has lots of energy and beautiful skin. She doesn't like foundation, so we used concealer only where her skin needs it.

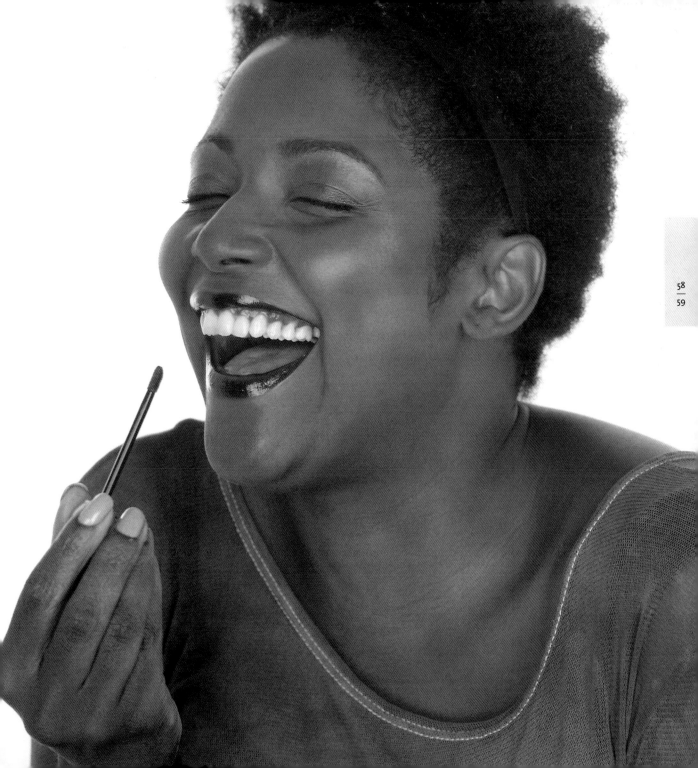

HOW TO CONCEAL UNDER-EYE PUFFINESS AND DARK CIRCLES

Sarah has beautiful eyes, but she suffers from allergies that often make them puffy and dark. To treat the puffiness, I recommend a gel-based eye cream at night to help keep swelling down. Remove the gel in the morning so you can apply concealer without it clumping.

I wanted to lighten up Sarah's eyes without using a lot of product to avoid that thick, cakey look. I also don't like using a lot of powder so I use a pigment-rich concealer. We used Jana (below) to illustrate how to use makeup to lighten under eyes that are dark but not puffy.

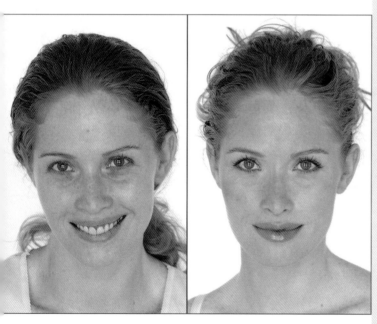

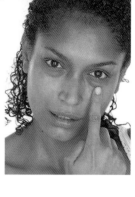

1 Apply moisturizer, primer, and concealer as usual, but not under the eyes.

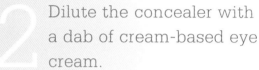

2 Dilute the concealer with a dab of cream-based eye cream.

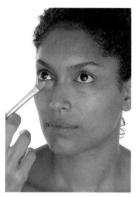

3 With your brush, cover only the dark parts under the eye and inside the socket by your nose. Covering the entire eye will only make the dark parts stay darker than the light parts that don't need to be lightened.

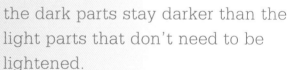

4 With clear translucent powder and brush, lightly coat the concealed part of the under eye.

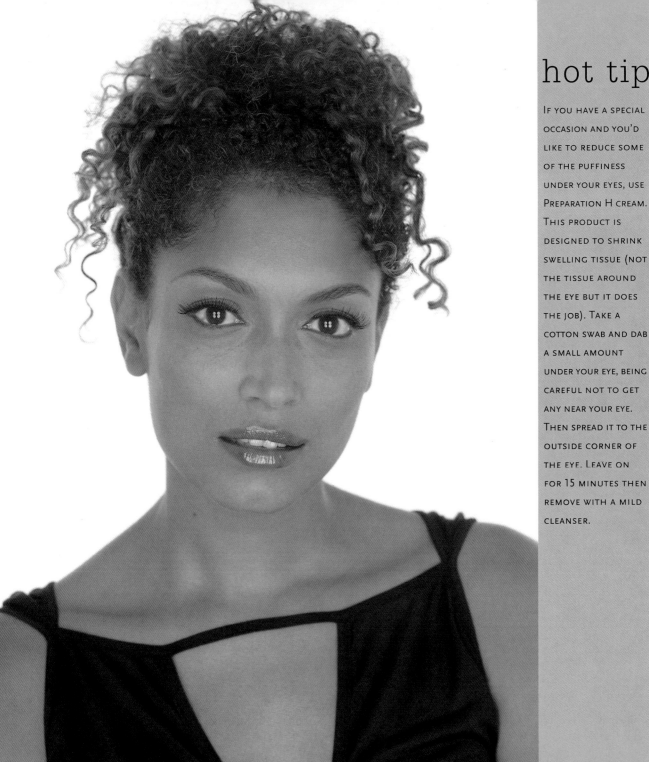

hot tip

IF YOU HAVE A SPECIAL OCCASION AND YOU'D LIKE TO REDUCE SOME OF THE PUFFINESS UNDER YOUR EYES, USE PREPARATION H CREAM. THIS PRODUCT IS DESIGNED TO SHRINK SWELLING TISSUE (NOT THE TISSUE AROUND THE EYE BUT IT DOES THE JOB). TAKE A COTTON SWAB AND DAB A SMALL AMOUNT UNDER YOUR EYE, BEING CAREFUL NOT TO GET ANY NEAR YOUR EYE. THEN SPREAD IT TO THE OUTSIDE CORNER OF THE EYF. LEAVE ON FOR 15 MINUTES THEN REMOVE WITH A MILD CLEANSER.

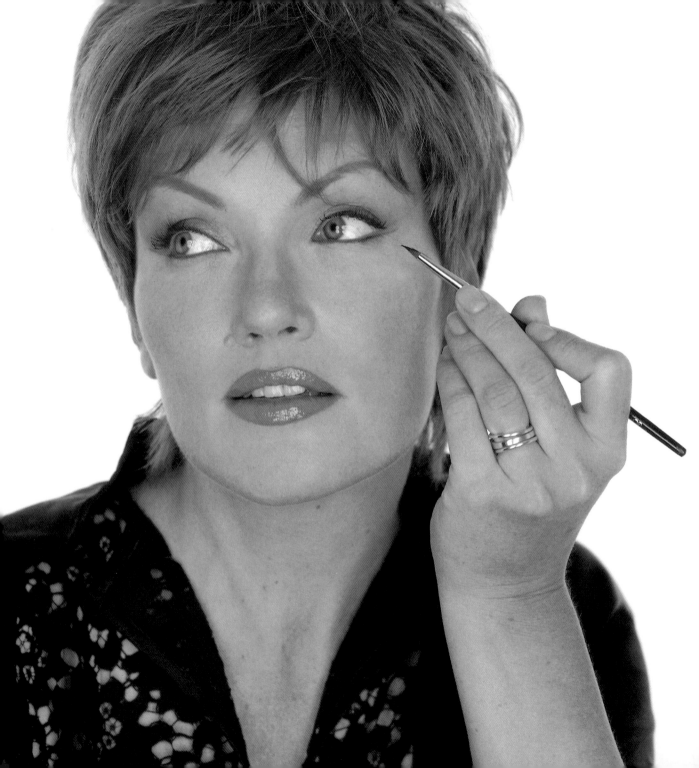

How to Add Contour to Enhance Your Best Features

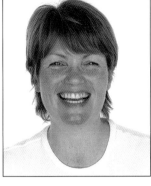

Wanda is a beautiful mother of two who loves to play with different looks. Her features really come alive with makeup.

Choose contour powder or cream stick by looking at your base and picking a color that is two or three shades darker. It's easy to find pressed powders for all colors of women today, and they're available in every price range.

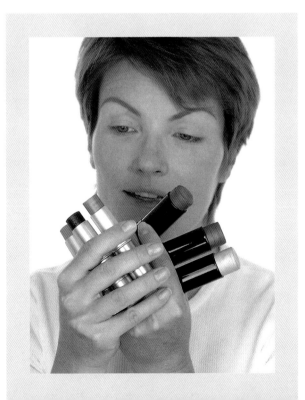

Contouring is a delicate procedure and should never look obvious. These are all meant to be illusions, slight differences that can change your look dramatically. So be sure to apply contour lightly. It's easier to add more than to have to rub your skin to get the brown streak off your cheek. Keep checking for the subtle difference in the mirror. If you only see dark powder, you've used too much. Believe me, you don't need a lot to give you a sunken look.

The rules of painting apply here also: where you use dark colors, features will recede. Where you use light colors, features will stand out. Putting dark powder on your cheekbones only makes them look flat. The trick is to put the darker color powder in the hollow of the cheek and add a lighter color to the actual cheekbone.

If you want your contouring to be very subtle, you can begin at step 7 on the following pages and use only powder.

1 Apply concealer and powder only where needed. Add blush to the apples of your cheeks only.

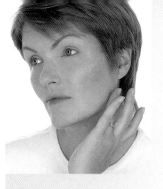

Do the same with the under-side of your jaw-bone, as pictured.

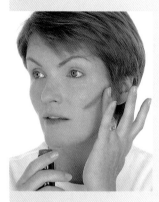

With your fingers, find the bottom part of your cheekbone. Apply a cream-based contour stick about a half an inch lower and draw a line from the back of your cheekbone to the middle of your cheek apple.

3 With a clean sponge lightly sweep downward and back toward your cheekbone, blending the color into the hollow of your cheek. Look in the mirror and locate the hollow of your cheeks. Suck them in if necessary to see the difference between your cheekbone and the hollow.

5 With a small synthetic brush, draw a thin line of color down the nose starting at the eye socket. Go as far as necessary to make the nose appear slightly thinner. You can also shade the sides of the nose by blending the color down the sides.

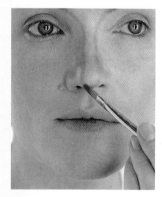

6 Blend all contour lines with a sponge. You shouldn't be able to see any lines. If you do, keep blending.

7 Now brush and sculpt the same areas with darker powder. This should also be almost invisible. I use a pressed,

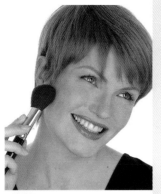

flat, nonshimmer powder designed for African-American women to contour my skin. Stay away from bronzers as you don't want any shimmer in the powder; the purpose here is to make the cheek look hollow, and shimmer is designed to highlight. Lay a fluffy, natural-hair brush on the powder and gently tap off all the excess. Sweep it lightly into the hollow and along the jaw line.

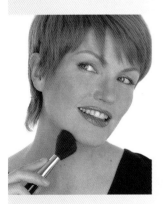

If you want your cheek-bones to appear bigger still, take a light pink blush that has some shimmer in it and gently sweep from your cheek apple to the bone right under the outside of your eye. You want to balance your cheeks with your hollows.

9 If you want a sun-kissed look, you can add a little of the darker powder to your fore-head and chin. Think about where the sun would naturally tan your face, and apply a gentle sweep of a slightly darker powder in those areas.

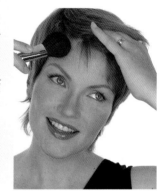

How to Thicken and Color Sparse Eyebrows

Patricia's eyebrows have a great shape but they're a little thin and sparse. With subtle filling and shaping you can see the difference a filled, shaped brow can make.

Great eyebrow pencils are hard to find. In order to apply enough wax to stick to the hairs you often end up with too much color on the eyebrow. Use a mostly wax pencil with only 35 to 50 percent pigment. When you apply color to the hair it appears darker, so select one that is slightly lighter than your natural color. Also, the oil in the skin will darken the powder and make the eyebrow look darker.

1 Fill in only the parts of your eyebrow that are sparse or where your hairs are lighter. Use the pencil in short, feathery movements, mimicking little brow hairs.

2 With a stiff brush and a complementary shadow color you can use the same motion to add some weight to the pencil wax that is already on your brow. Make sure that the base of the brow shadow is a color complementary to your hair color. Use a brow brush (an old toothbrush will work) to blend all the colors together and separate the hairs.

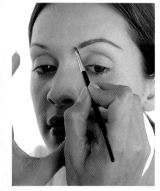

3 Add a little translucent powder to the brow and continue to brush up and out, giving your brow a nice shape. You can set it with clear mascara or a little hairspray on your brow brush.

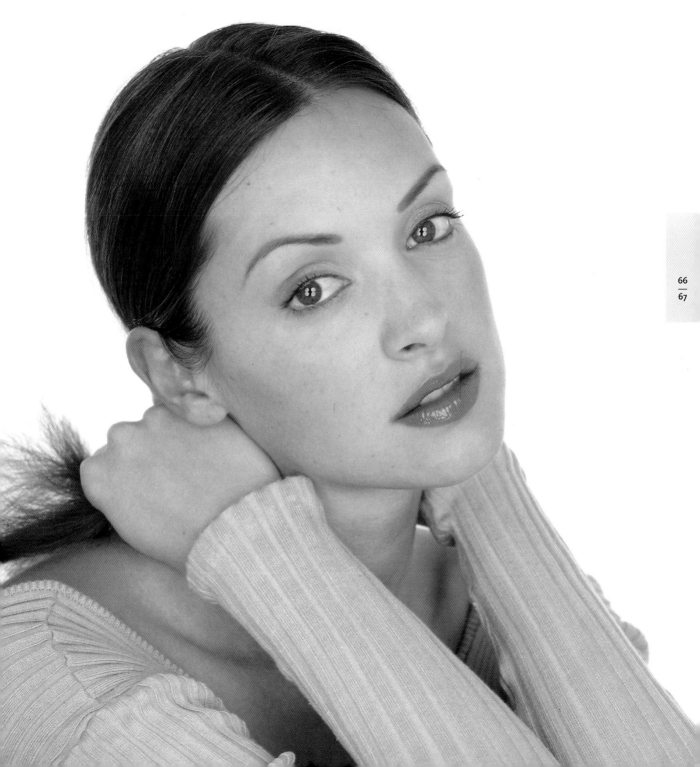

HOW TO MAKE YOUR EYES LOOK BIGGER

Alise has great, almond-shaped eyes. We just wanted to make them appear larger so they are in better proportion to her other features.

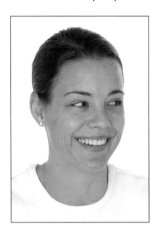

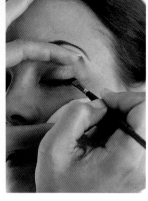

1 After lining the eye, take the liner to the middle of the lid (just above your iris) and make that section slightly thicker. Then taper the line toward the inside and outside corners, so it won't be obvious.

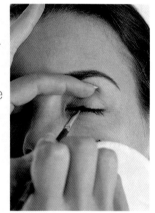

2 Add your normal shadow, always keeping that middle part a little thicker and more intense.

3 When you add mascara remember to concentrate on those center lashes, using a second coat to make them appear longer. This will open up the eye and make it rounder.

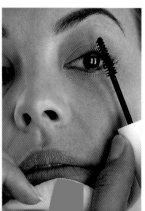

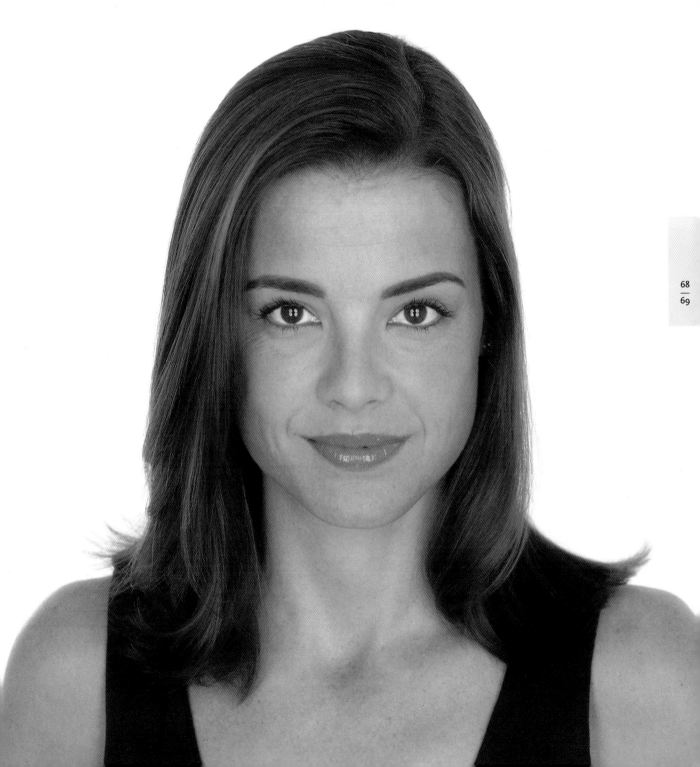

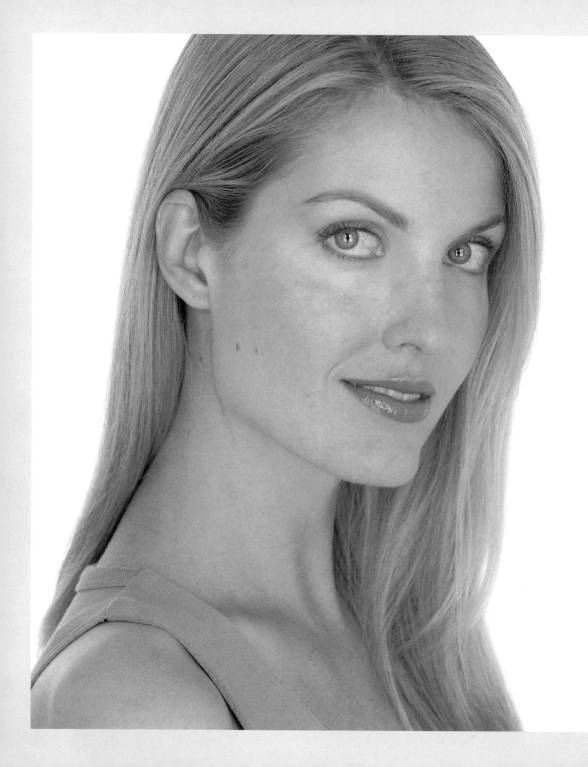

HOW TO USE MAKEUP TO LIFT YOUR EYES

Melanie has big blue eyes, but she feels they should be lifted slightly. If your hair and skin are light like hers, it's important to use a taupe or brown liner. You don't want the liner to be obvious.

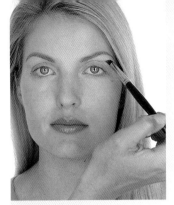

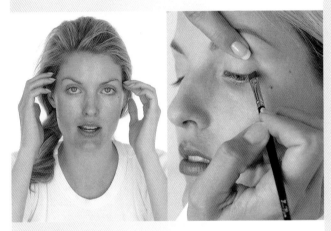

1 As you line the eye, gently drag the liner up at the corners. Then smudge the second coat of liner up and in toward the center of the eye.

Using a shadow only a few shades darker than your skin tone, apply from the center of the eye just above the iris and move directly out. Be careful not to follow the crease or you will create a socket that will make the eye turn down again. You want to create a gentle shadow that seems to pull the eye up.

3 Use an eyelash curler to lift those corner lashes. Use mascara but avoid the lashes at the very outside of the eye where they tend to grow down. Leave those last lashes bare and give the middle and inner lashes two coats.

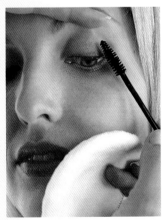

HOW TO OPEN UP CLOSE-SET EYES

My eyes are very close set in relation to my cheekbones.

1 As I line my eyes, I wing the line slightly out and up. Then I add a slight shading to the outside corners of my eyes. This draws the eye out.

2 Using a color only a few shades darker than my skin, I smudge that outside line farther out and up.

3 Then I apply shadow in the crease from the top of my iris straight out, not following the downward curve of my brow bone.

4 On the top of my lid I put a lighter shade with shine so it reflects light and makes my eyes stand out.

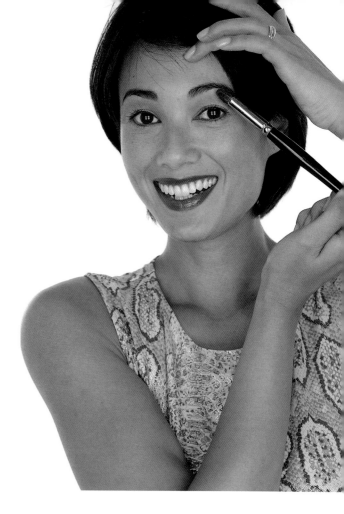

HOW TO CREATE THE ILLUSION OF DEPTH FOR FLAT EYES

Some women have either no eye crease or very flat eyes. Creating the illusion of depth is easy if you use subtle colors that are only a few shades darker than your skin color. I wanted to give Lisa a subtle, yet more deep-set eye.

1. After doing your invisible liner (page 49), line the eyes again with wet, flat liner.

2. With a color similar to your lid, sweep from lash line to brow line.

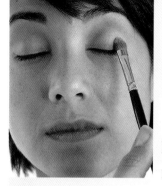

Using a color several shades lighter, take a natural-hair brush and dot color directly on the lid where your iris is. This will create a lighter lid and make it stand out more.

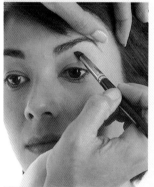

Open your eye and look straight into a mirror. Take a soft pointed natural-hair brush up about 1/4 inch above where your lashes end (which is also about 1/4 inch below your eyebrow). You don't want to make the eye smaller so keep this color above your actual crease line. Sweep a clean line of slightly darker shade into that crease. Keep blending and pulling up and out to keep it lifted.

5. Using a lighter color with a slight shimmer, sweep shadow along the top of the brow bone.

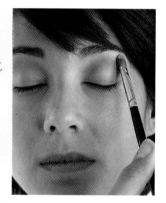

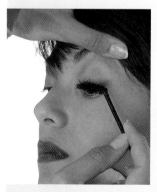

Don't forget mascara. It will further open the eye up and create more intensity.

HOW TO CREATE THE AUDREY HEPBURN EYE WITH INDIVIDUAL LASHES

Audrey Hepburn made the lifted liner and false eyelash famous. It's much easier to achieve than you might think. Brenda, an actress and mom, has round eyes and likes to make them look more almond. This is a great way to do a quick dramatic look, or use lighter brown to make your eyes look sleeker, more almond shaped.

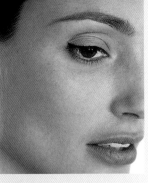

1 With a shadow color slightly lighter than your lid color, sweep from lash root to brow bone.

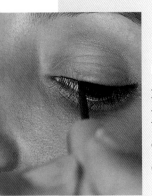

2 Line your eye with pencil liner as shown for the basic face, then with a liquid liner go over that line with a thicker line. Concentrate on keeping the line very close to the lashes at the inside of the eye.

3 While lifting the brow with your ring finger, extend the line out and up from the outside part of your eye. You can fill this in slightly to make a darker, thicker tail but make sure you keep it pointed and tapered at the end.

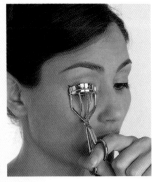

4 Curl your lashes and apply two coats of black mascara.

5 False eyelashes come in clumps of three; glue four of these to the last group of lashes on the outer sides of your eyes. You don't need to add more mascara. You can also use a full line of lashes for a more dramatic effect.

6 This look can be even more reminiscent of Audrey Hepburn if you thicken and darken your eyebrows.

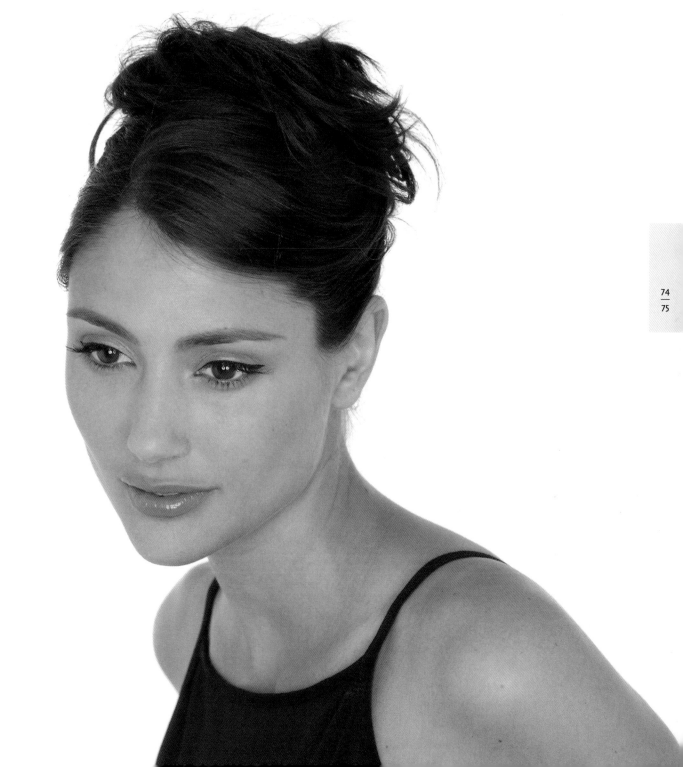

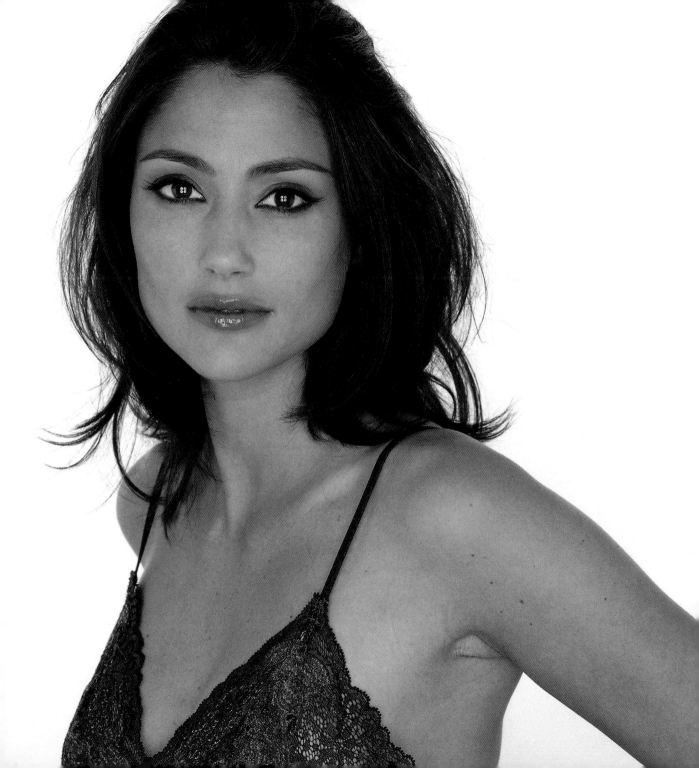

How to Create the Smokey Eye

This is another easy dramatic look. I wanted to show you the difference between this and the Hepburn eye. See how this look makes Brenda's eyes even more almond shaped.

1 After doing your invisible liner, line the entire eye on the skin. Flare out on the outside corner if you want a sleek, modern Cleopatra look.

2 Use a flat, wet liner to add intensity, extending it past the corners.

3 With a dark black, brown, or gray shadow and a small smudging brush, line the entire eye, smudging the wet liner and pencil. Blending is key because you don't want to see the pencil line at all. Pencils are mostly wax, and when wax heats up from the skin, it tends to smear. Smudging your pencil line with shadow alleviates this problem and makes your eye appear softer, more natural. It lasts much longer, too.

4 Using a color two to three shades darker than your skin, contour the crease of your eye. Blend and pull the shadow out to the corners.

5 Curl your lashes and apply two coats of black mascara.

6 For an even more dramatic look you can attach individual false lashes to the outside corners—or all over.

Keep in mind that if your eyes are this intense you should keep your lips a lighter shade. I used a neutral pencil liner and a clear pink/ brown gloss on Brenda so her eyes really pop.

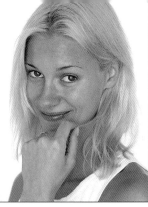

How to Complement Your Eyes with Color

Simple color matches are good for certain eye and hair colors; there are ways to work with color that can help with different problems. For instance, if you have redness or dark circles under your eyes, you should keep blue and gray tones away from around the eye. These colors will only accentuate the darkness, even if you've covered it with concealer. On the other hand, if you have blue or green eyes and you want them to stand out, use a red- or orange-based color, because red tones tend to pull the yellow out of the iris and showcase blue or green eyes. These might seem like complicated rules, but once you're familiar with the tones and notice what happens when you apply certain colors, it will become fun to experiment. If you love blue eye shadow then by all means use it! What's important is that you blend the blue in a way that high-lights the eye, not the shadow.

Elizabeth has beautiful eyes to begin with, but she'd like the blue to pop a little more. Choosing complementary colors can make your eyes really stand out.

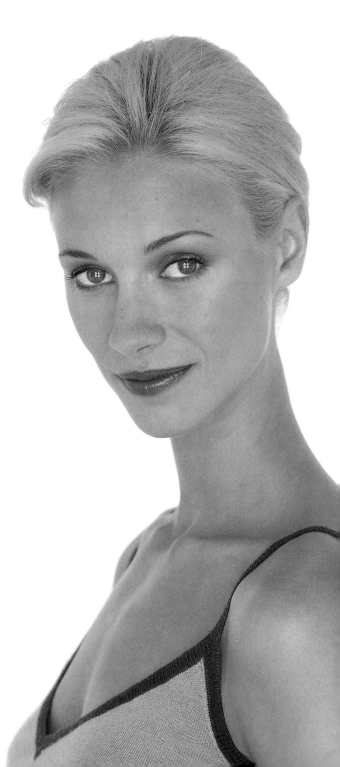

1 Sweep a color close to your own lid color or translucent powder from lash line to brow line.

2 Do your invisible liner, and apply the wet liner in a color that complements your eye color. This is usually a red- or orange-based color. It shouldn't actually be red or orange but the color should have that base tone. Red cancels out yellow in the iris so your true iris color will stand out more.

3 Blend a sheer version of the color you used for the liner into the crease of your eye. Remember to keep your eye open and put the brush directly above your lashes while the eye is open. This will keep the crease high and avoid making the eye seem smaller.

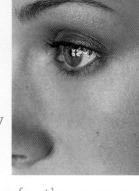

4 You can either use a lighter shade for directly on top of the lid or use the sheer color that you use for the crease. The latter is a better look for evening.

5 You can make your lips intense or keep them natural with this shadow style. If you like a strong lip, use the same tone you used on your eyelids, and it will highlight your eyes even more.

HOW TO MAKE YOUR MAKEUP SWEATPROOF

Audra works out and swims regularly, and she has oily skin. She likes to have some color on her face when she works out or swims. I recommend using gel- or liquid-based blushes and bronzers. The key to making gel- or liquid-based makeup look natural is to find a color that closely resembles the color of your skin when you naturally blush or tan.

1 Use concealer only where you really need it, allowing your skin to breathe while you work out or play.

2 With a small sponge (you can use your fingertips, but the gel will temporarily stain your fingers so I recommend a sponge), apply a gel/liquid-based blush to the apples of your cheeks, gently rubbing it in. Make sure it's where you want it, because it's going to stay put!

3 Pucker your lips like you're giving a big kiss and dot some right in the middle. Smack your lips together or use your finger to fine-tune the lip coverage. Now

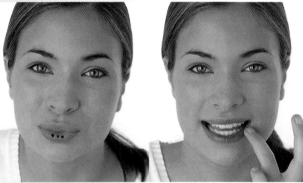

you have perfectly colored lips that will last all through the day. For an evening look, you can add lip gloss.

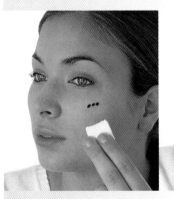
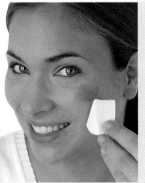

USING FALSE LASHES

False lashes are coming back in style, perhaps because using "false hair"—wigs, hair weaves, and falls—is becoming more popular, too. Just as with wigs, the quality of the lashes is better and they look more like real lashes than the old ones. I am often asked if I can do lashes myself, as most women think it's too difficult to apply them. I want you to see how easy it is to use single, clump, or full false lashes. If it's your first time I recommend lashes in little tufts of three lashes in one root.

1 Curl your natural lashes and apply one coat of mascara. Use a lash separator.

2 Holding the false lashes with tweezers, dip the root in the glue. I use black glue if I'm using dark liner and clear if I'm keeping the makeup light. Blow on it for a few seconds to make the glue tacky so you won't have to hold it on the lash very long to set it.

3 Close one eye and simply place the false lash directly above your last outside lash.

4 Apply four or five more tufts, from the outside in.

5 You can add one more coat of mascara if you are doing a very dramatic eye. Or leave them bare for a more natural look.

Once you get used to keeping your eye closed and placing the lashes down you can try a full set of lashes. They come in every hair color now, even blond and red. You don't have to save them for special events—you can use them anytime.

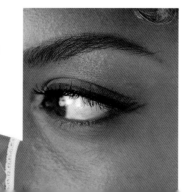

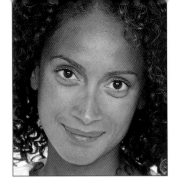

How to Apply Makeup without Brushes

Marita travels more than anyone I know. She wanted to learn how to apply makeup in two minutes without a brush or a mirror. When I'm on the run and I just want some soft shading, I use cream shadows, blushes, and lipstick, so I can do my face by touch alone.

1 Apply concealer with your fingers. Then rub a cream shadow that's a few shades lighter than your skin tone directly on the top of your eyelid. You can leave it just above the lashes or extend it up to the brow bone.

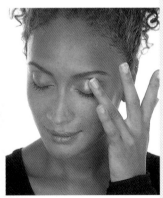

2 Using a cream or stick blush, gently dot on the apple of your cheeks and blend with your fingers. Feel for your cheekbone and make sure you're not pulling the color too close to your temples.

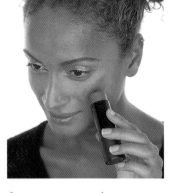

3 With a lipstick or pot gloss dab color on your lips using your fingers to spread it out and make it smooth.

4 Use mascara, or just leave your eyelashes bare.

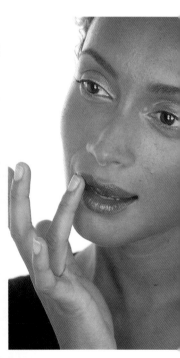

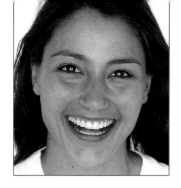

HOW TO MAKE YOUR LIPS LOOK FULLER

Lining the natural ridge of your lip, as opposed to the color ridge, as I've shown, can make your lips look bigger, but if you want even fuller lips, follow these steps.

1   Line the natural ridge but don't fill in the lip with pencil.

2   Fill in the lip with a lipstick that is one or two shades lighter than your pencil (I'm not talking about a red liner with light pink in the middle—that never looks natural. Just a few shades lighter will give you the illusion of a fuller middle lip).

3   After you've filled the lip in, use your ring finger and dab a little cream or white dry eye shadow onto the middle of both your top and bottom lip. Gently press your lips together to soften the shadow. This highlights the middle even more. Remember, if you can see the shadow, you've used too much. It is an illusion and should not be obvious.

4   If you want a glossy lip, now is the time to pat a little gloss in the middle of the lip, on top of the shadow, and gently press your lips together. Don't put the gloss all the way to the edges— it will start to run and look messy.

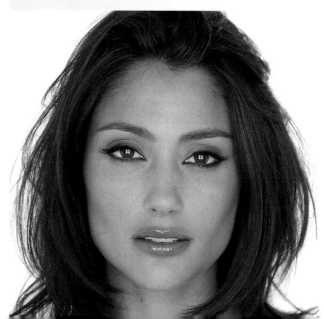

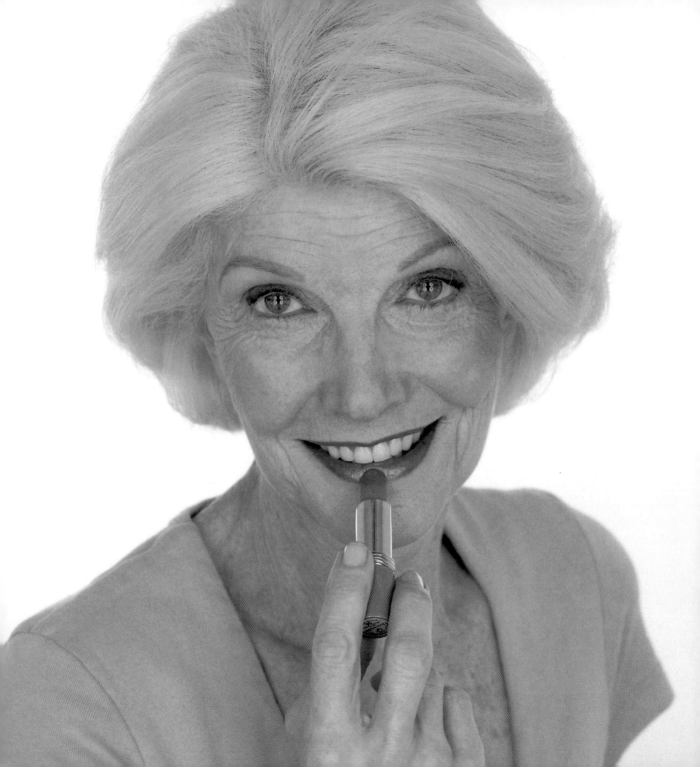

THE ANTI-FEATHER LIP

Gloria is an active woman who wants to put her lipstick on only once a day, and she doesn't want to worry about it bleeding into fine lines around her mouth. Many lipsticks contain silicone now to avoid this, but silicone tends to be very drying and your lips will need constant moisture.

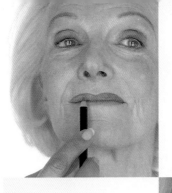

Fill in the entire lip with pencil.

1 Do your basic face.

2 Cover your entire lip, just over the natural ridge line, with concealer.

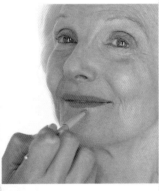

With lip liner, line your natural lip ridge (not the color line).

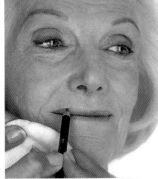

5 Lay a tissue separated in half on top of your lips and cover your lips with a light dusting of loose powder.

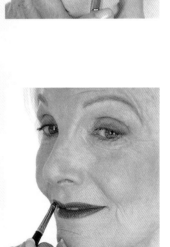

6 Coat your lips with lipstick and off you go!

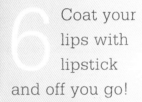

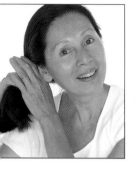

THE FIVE-MINUTE MAKEOVER

Kedaki is a real estate agent. She always has fifteen things going on at once so she only has five minutes to do her makeup.

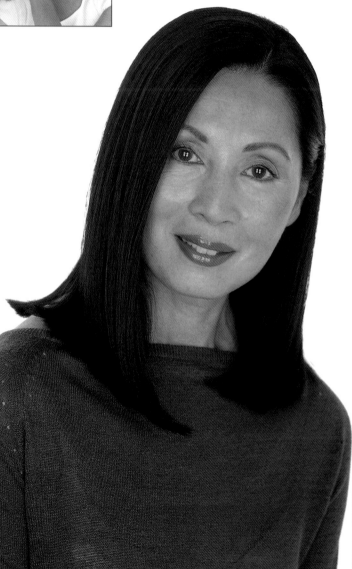

1 Moisturize right out of the shower.

2 Apply primer to your face.

3 Use concealer only where you need it.

4 Use powder on the areas where you used concealer.

5 Add cream blush to the apples of your cheeks.

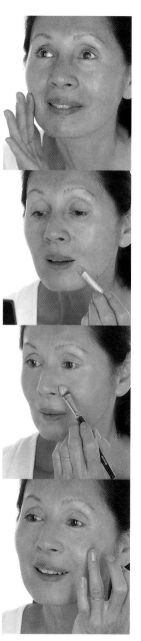

6   Fill in your eyebrows.

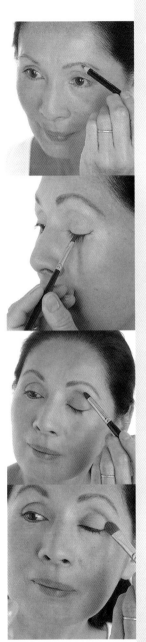

7   Do your invisible liner, and smudge the line while the liner is still wet.

8   Apply shadow two shades darker than your skin to the crease of your eye.

9   Apply shadow one shade lighter than your skin on the top of the lid and on the brow bone.

10   Apply one or two coats of mascara.

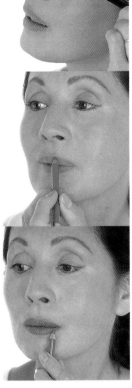

11   Line the lips and fill in with liner.

12   Finish with lip gloss.

Truly five minutes.
Each step flows
right into
the next one.

THE THREE-PRODUCT, THREE-MINUTE EVENING MAKEOVER

To take this into evening with only three products and three more minutes:

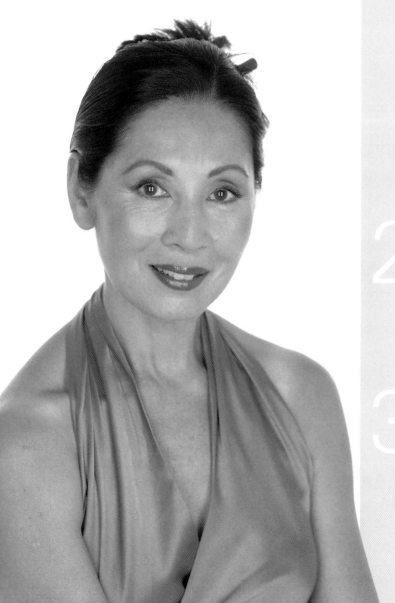

1 Use a black pencil liner to line the top of the eye. Smudge the line with a cotton swab. Use the leftover liner on the swab to smudge under the bottom lashes.

2 Dab your lipstick on the apple of your cheek. Rub up and out to blend the color.

3 Use the same lipstick on your lips. Add gloss for extra glamour.

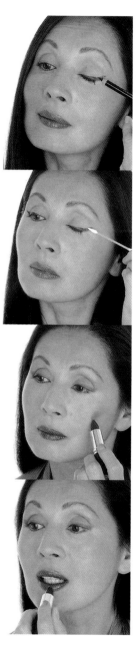

4 Apply mascara. Then twist your hair around and secure with a hair stick or barrette.

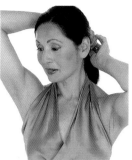

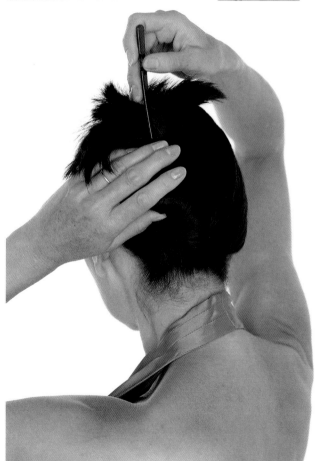

a

new

you

in

just

five

minutes

wedding and event makeup

Most women find it frustrating to transform their makeup from day to evening or for different occasions. Andrea's routine must be fast and fabulous for all of her work-related events.

EVENING MAKEUP

When working for catalogs we have to change from a day look to an evening look within minutes. I have pared this down slightly so that a few products in your little makeup bag will enable you to change your look according to your mood and the occasion. A little planning goes a long way when you're talking about changing your daytime look to an evening dazzler.

1 Determine what you're going to wear as your office or daytime attire and if there is one item you can change to make the outfit more appropriate for an evening occasion. If you're wearing a dark suit, for instance, perhaps you can simply change the shirt or camisole underneath.

2 If you know in advance what color dress or shirt you will be wearing and also what type of light you will be in, you can customize your kit and change your makeup accordingly.

3 Keep the following items in your bag: a darker pigmented lipstick, a brown or black crayon-type liner, and pressed powder. In just a couple of minutes you can refresh your powder, eyeliner, and lipstick (which you can also use as an instant blush, blending it with your fingertip).

4 Do your five-minute makeover (pages 88–89).

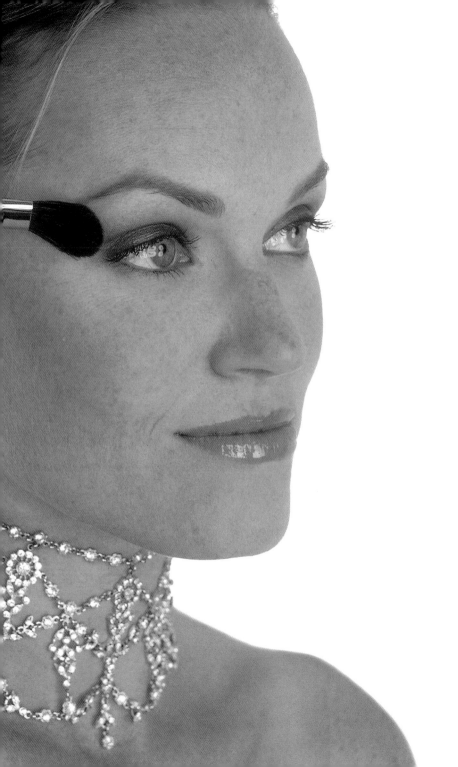

WEDDING MAKEUP

One of the most important special occasions is your wedding day. You can't take any chances with it. I love doing makeup for brides. I always start by telling brides two things, whether they're hiring a professional or doing their own makeup: 1) I want a woman to feel like a twelve-year-old girl who just got out of bed: clean, fresh, and without obvious makeup. You don't want to shock your groom with a look he's never seen before. You should feel beautiful and comfortable on your big day. If a bride asks me to do something I do it. Even if I don't completely agree. 2) Look in books and magazines for pictures of makeup or hair that you like, even it's just the lip color or eye color. You can use these as you play with your makeup yourself or as a guide for the professional makeup artist. You should always do at least one consultation with the artist before the big day.

1 After doing your basic face, use a gel-based cheek color before your powder blush. This layering will keep you glowing from the inside and will add dimension for photos.

2 Don't use a lot of contouring. You don't want to change your face too much. If you want a little contouring, at least make sure that you can't see the powder.

3 Use the gel-based blush on your lips before you apply your liner for the same reason as the blush. Then do the anti-feather lip (see page 85) for long-lasting color. Go easy on the gloss because it will reflect in photographs.

4 This is a time for more powder than I usually recommend. It should look good in pictures but still look natural in real life. Make sure you use only clear translucent powder around your creases or eyes. Use colored powder only where your face is flat.

5 To make your eyes more dramatic, refer to pages 74–75 for adding individual lashes.

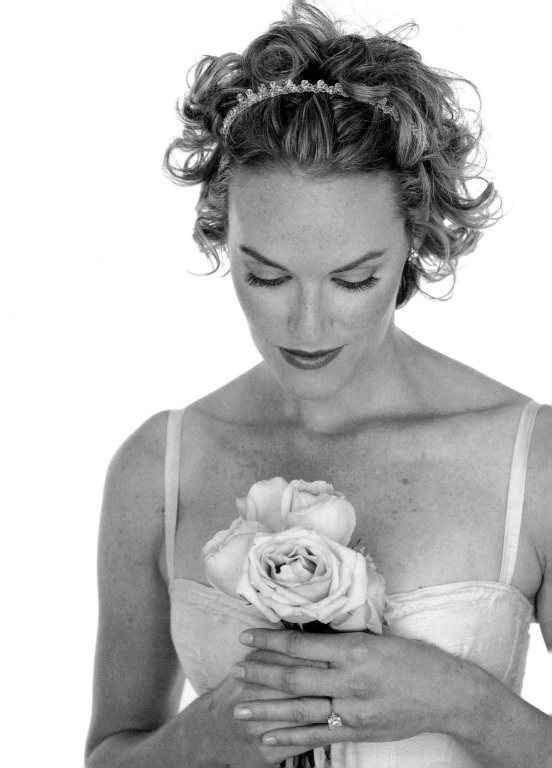

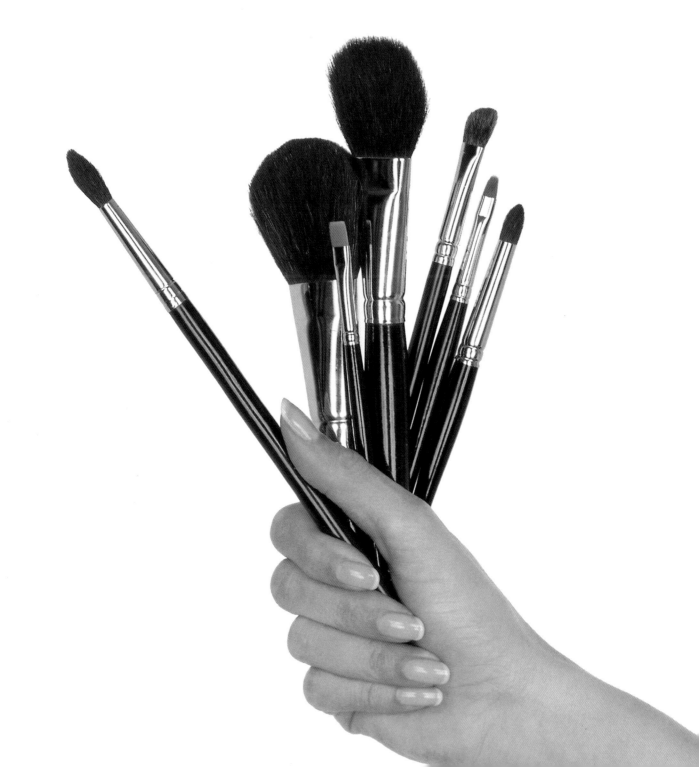

your brushes

Over the years I have become an expert on brushes and makeup tools. Some people think that any brush will suffice when it comes to applying makeup. That couldn't be further from the truth. Fortunately, great makeup brushes are available, but the down side is that the good ones don't come cheap. However, if you care for them correctly they can last a lifetime, so you might want to invest in a few. I have brushes from ten years ago that I still use every day. I have paid full, high prices but have also found some of my very favorite brushes at discount prices. I will show you how to tell a good brush from a mediocre one, at any price level, and how to care for them once you make the investment.

NATURAL VERSUS SYNTHETIC

Natural brushes are made of animal hair, and synthetic brushes are made of man-made hair. Big, natural brushes, such as a powder or cheek color brush, are usually made of goat or pony hair. Brushes for eye color or a shorter haired brush can be made of sable, goat, or squirrel. Most of the smaller brushes are made of sable. This is usually the softest of the hairs but also the most expensive.

Natural bristles are absorbent. Think about this when you are applying makeup. These brushes soak up color and then hold on to it. This is great when you want to add a small amount of color and need to be able to blend without adding more color than you need. Using these brushes for creams is not a great idea because as they absorb the product, they don't release it easily. When you're trying to put a sheer coat of concealer cream on and you have to keep pressing the brush on your skin, the concealer is pushed back into the bristles. This is when you should use a synthetic brush. It doesn't absorb the product, so it can release easily without even bending the bristles. Knowing this simple fact can help you recognize a useful brush, no matter what the price is.

THE RIGHT BRUSH

In all brushes, you want to look for smooth, unfrayed hairs. The bristles should be evenly cut and thick enough so that when you gently bend them, they splay thickly and evenly. When you brush your face with them, they should feel soft and gentle, almost like little feathers running across your face. You should be able to run your fingers around the bristles from the handle to the tips without pulling any hairs out.

The hairs of a brush can be attached to their wands in many different ways. The hairs on the cheapest brushes are simply glued onto the wand, and then a barrel is put on top. The best brushes have hairs that are first tied together, then glued to the wand; the metal barrel is pressed flat around the hairs, making it look like it was smashed. If your brushes are in a perfect round barrel you know that they are either glued or glued and tied, so you should be careful not to get the base of the barrel wet when washing them. If you see an expensive brush that you like, you should ask how it is made before buying it.

SIX GREAT BRUSHES EVERYONE SHOULD HAVE

There are many brushes on the market and once you get used to shopping for them and doing your own makeup you will know what you need. I like having lots of brushes when I'm doing someone else's makeup, because I never know what I'm going to need. But for my own makeup, I use only the six brushes described below.

1 A camouflage brush. A synthetic brush, it should be thin, flat, and tightly bound. The tip of the brush should be rounded or slightly pointed. You want this brush to be thin so the product won't collect in the center hairs. You want it to be flat because you don't want it to hold too much product or you will have to press hard on your face to get the product off the brush.

2 A synthetic brush for applying clear translucent powder on top of concealer. This should be a thin brush with slightly

long bristles. It should feel like silk as you brush it across your face.

3 A synthetic brush for eyeliner. This brush should be thin, tightly bound, and perfectly straight across the tip. It should be a quarter-inch wide so that you can use it to press your eyeliner into the base of your eyelashes. If it is much wider you will have a hard time getting it into the inside corner of the eye. I don't recommend a pointed, natural-hair brush for eyeliner, because it is hard to keep that line straight when doing it yourself. Also for most women, the flat eyeliner used against the eyelashes is the easiest and most natural way to highlight and define the eye.

4 A natural, angled eye shadow brush for your crease and lid. It should have a slightly pointed tip for directing your crease shadow smoothly and precisely. The flatter edge will give you control as you apply color to your lid. This brush is useful for sweeping on small amounts of color, blending as you go.

5 A large, natural, long-bristled brush for face powder. It should be tightly bound, with a round top. Use this for just the apple of your cheek, not for smearing bronzer or other colors all over your face.

6 A lip brush. This can be made of either natural or synthetic hair. I happen to like a lip brush made with natural hair because I like to control the application, adding little bits of color at a time, rather than having the lipstick lay on the top of a synthetic brush and then pushing it around the lip. These are usually not the most expensive brushes in your kit so you can experiment to see which one you like better. I like a semi-rounded tip, not too pointed but not straight. If the

point is too sharp it will be very hard to give yourself a perfect line without a great deal of practice, unless you have an incredibly steady hand. I don't recommend a square-tipped lip brush either, for the obvious reason that you need some point to do your top ridge.

CARING FOR YOUR BRUSHES

First you buy a great brush and then you have to care for it like a fine piece of china. But if you follow some simple guidelines your brushes can last a long time. I wash my brushes like a fanatic after each use. I have to because I use my brushes on different women every day. You probably don't use your brushes on other people's faces like I do, but even so, you have oils and germs on your skin, as well as all the makeup products you're using. This means dirty brushes. While you don't have to wash all of your brushes every day, I would recommend cleaning your camouflage brush every day, even just with a makeup/baby wipe. I wash my color brushes once a week, using the following procedure.

1. Run the brush under warm water trying not to get the metal barrel wet. This is important: water that invades the barrel weakens the glue.

2. With a mild soap or shampoo gently rub the hairs between your fingers. Work the soap into the base of the brush but not into the barrel.

3. Under tepid running water and with the same gentle rubbing motion, rinse the soap and dirt out of the brush until you feel that the hairs are squeaky clean.

4. Gently press your fingers together to flatten the hairs into the brush's original shape. You can wrap a towel around the brush to press the excess water out, but do not rub the brush into the towel. This will only fray the hairs and eventually break them off.

5. Set the brush down on a flat surface that has an edge, like a table or countertop. Put the handle and barrel on the edge with the hairs extending over the edge. You can lay the towel on top of the handles to keep the brushes from falling over the edge. The reason you don't want to put the brushes straight up in a cup is because the water from the hairs will run down into the barrel and weaken the glue. Your brushes should dry overnight. If they don't, you can use the cool setting of a blow-dryer. Just don't splay the hairs out as you dry it.

This process can add life to your brushes. Some of my oldest brushes are in the same shape as my new brushes.

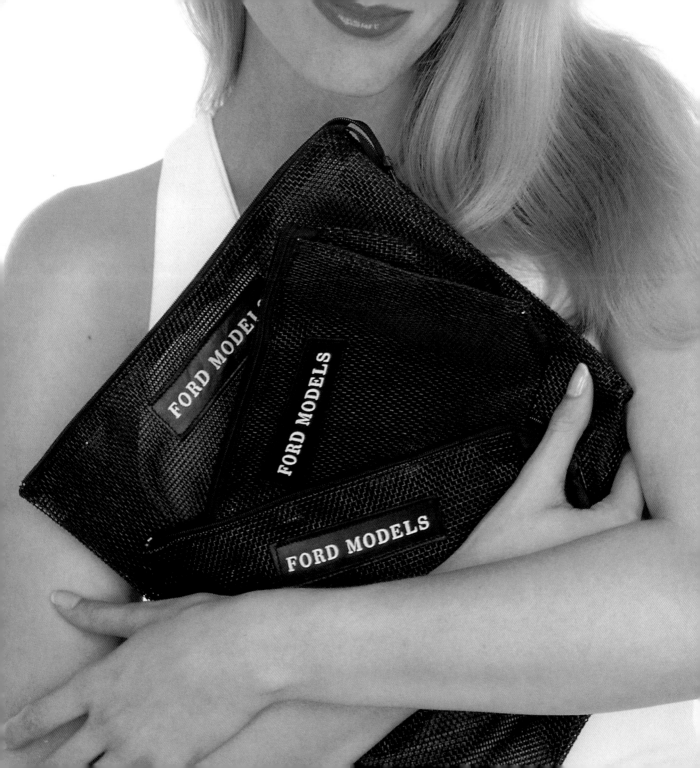

bring your bag

How many products do you keep in your makeup bag? If you're like most women, models included, you have too much stuff. Do you use all of it? Do you know which products have many different uses? Do you know the shelf life of all your products? This section is dedicated to cleaning out that makeup bag and stocking it with products that are multi-functional. I'll also explain which products need to be replaced and how often. Makeup packaging usually indicates its expiration date. The most important expiration dates to remember are those of the products that go onto your eyes; if they are old or contaminated, they can cause irritation or infection.

I always travel light, often taking along no more than a carry-on bag or two. That means paring down to the bare necessities. When working, models usually have skilled makeup artists on hand, but in case we don't, having our favorite makeup with us can make or break a job.

YOUR MAKEUP BAG

In my makeup bag, I keep a small jar of moisturizer, primer, eye cream, eyelash curler, and mascara. Everything else is optional. Next, I pack concealer, translucent powder, and a cream blush. For my eyes I include a brow pencil, and brown and black eye pencils, which can be used alone or with shadows. The shadows I pack are a creamy light yellow or pink, a caramel color, a soft brown, and a dark brown or black. For lips, a neutral light-brown pencil, a soft pink or brown color, and a gloss with some shimmer.

Let's look at what's in your makeup bag and see how old it is. Mascara has a shelf life of one to four months. As soon as mascara is opened and exposed to air it picks up bacteria. When the wand is put back into the tube, this bacteria multiplies. I keep an extra new one on hand and always write the date on the cap so I can keep track.

Foundation is also a prime place for bacteria. You may not get an infection but it could be causing some reactions that result in skin eruptions. The shelf life of foundation is about six months. Try to keep it in a cool place and always shake your foundation before using.

Your Travel Bag

There are some easy, basic steps to combat the jet-lag look. Always carry your "travel bag," a bag designed for comfort and relaxation to keep packed and ready to go at a moment's notice. Here's what I include: earplugs, extra socks, a paperback book, a Walkman and my two favorites tapes, lip balm, hand cream, an eye mask, herbal remedies for colds and flu, eyedrops, pain relievers, a scented candle with a cover, toothbrush and paste, a deck of cards, gum, and a big bottle of water. Now, no matter how long it takes me to get somewhere, I have what I need to keep me comfortable.

Once I get to a hotel room I immediately light my candle so the smell is familiar. You'd be surprised how important a scent you love is to your mood. If I have room in my bag I also bring my favorite pillowcase. This again is about familiarity.

Your Good Night Bag

I devote this bag to products I keep by my bedside and use before I go to sleep. It always contains an unscented lotion for hands and elbows, lip balm, cuticle softener, and, in winter, an alpha-hydroxy peppermint foot lotion.

Buying Makeup on the Road

If you've lost or forgotten your makeup bag and you're desperate for a quick face, there are four basic, inexpensive products that can be purchased at any drugstore.

1 A concealer that is the same tone (yellow or pink) as your under-skin. Turn over your wrist and look at the color. This is a place that rarely sees the sun. It will be either a yellow/green tone or a blue/pink/white tone. With your ring finger, warm the concealer up, and with tiny, gentle pats cover any blemishes on your face or circles under your eyes. Remember that since you won't have powder, you'll want the concealer to be completely sheer.

2 Next you'll need blush. Choose the blush the same way as the concealer. If your base skin color is yellow, keep your blush a warm pink. If your base is blue/white, make it a cool pink. These will blend well without streaking. A cream blush will eliminate the need for a brush, but you can use a cotton ball. You can also use a little of the blush for the crease of your eye. With a small amount on your ring finger, pat the center of the eye and smear out.

3 Mascara, which can be used like eyeliner. Apply the mascara and slightly smudge the wand on the root line directly above the eyelash. Actually try to make a slightly messy line—this is meant to look like smudged eyeliner. With a damp cotton swab, smudge the line of the black or gray color around the lashes. It's a tricky process, but it looks like you did it on purpose if you're careful.

4 Last, choose a lip color that is sheer or frosted so you don't have to use a liner. This will keep the lip soft and smudge-free. With only four products and a cotton swab you have saved yourself from a barefaced disaster!

your hair

Whether your hair is thick and curly or fine and straight, there are simple steps you can take to make your hair look more beautiful. I will show you how to make baby-fine hair look like it has tons of volume and how to turn frizzy, curly, unruly hair into beautiful, soft curls. I'll show you how you can completely change your look by getting a new haircut or using different accessories. I will teach you how to take care of your hair and judge products based on the ingredients in them. The hair industry is flooded with new products; we'll wade through them and I'll help you decide which products are right for you. We will also do a color correction on someone who has had one too many blond colors put into her hair and wants to return to her natural color with an easy at-home coloring.

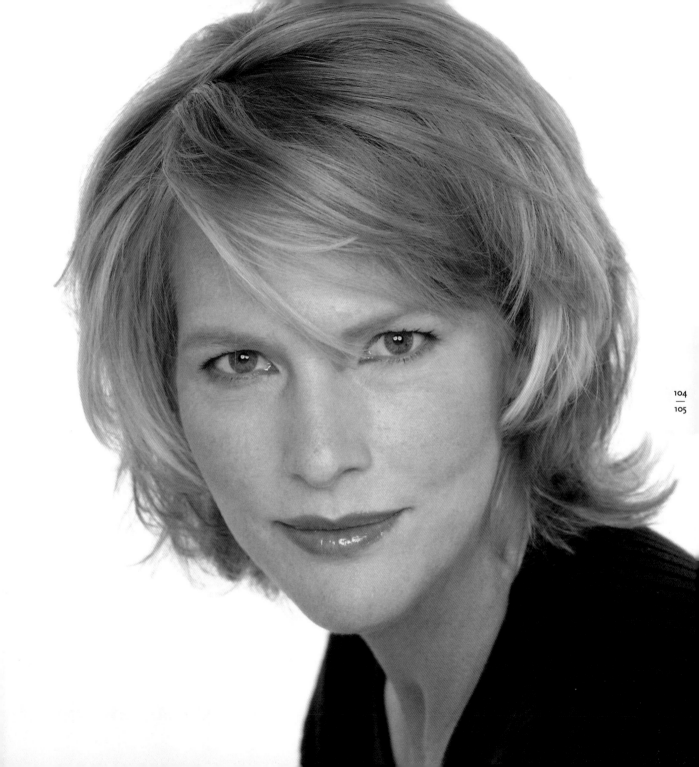

you
should only
use
shampoo
if your
hair is
truly dirty.

daily maintenance

Keeping your hair in good condition is extremely important. Being a model has been very hard on my hair. Stylists are only concerned with making my hair look good for a specific shoot; if a client wants my curly hair to be straight that day, the stylist has no choice but to fry it and make it straight. So I spend a great deal of time fixing my damaged hair.

SHAMPOOING

I think that Americans are suds-obsessed. We want that squeaky-clean feeling and assume that it only happens if we have lots of suds. But these suds remove all of the natural sebum from your scalp, so you should only use shampoo if your hair is truly dirty. I wash my hair with shampoo only once a week. The other days I wash it with conditioner. I put it in and scrub as I would with shampoo and then rinse. It cleans mildly, without stripping the hair completely, which is especially important if you have dry hair. If you have oily hair, use a mild shampoo that doesn't contain silicone (see the box on page 121). If you do shampoo your hair every day, don't

massage your scalp too aggressively. This will activate the oil glands and you'll end up with oily hair at the end of the day. I would also try some of the brands found in health food stores. They usually have less stripping detergents and some of the botanicals can be very therapeutic for your scalp.

CONDITIONING

Although hot oil treatments make hair silky, the oil molecule is too large to actually penetrate the hair shaft, so I use two different conditioners: a deep placenta and protein conditioner to rebuild the shaft after coloring, and a deep hydrating conditioner that comes in a mask and an in-shower conditioner. The protein makes the hair stronger and more tolerant of heat. If your hair is oily, use conditioner only on the ends.

Of course, it's not possible to completely repair your hair once it has been truly damaged. The only solution is to cut it off. Regular eighth-of-an-inch trims will keep your hair from thinning out due to broken ends. I get my hair trimmed every other month. If it seems dry or split, I just get a trim. If you're trying to grow your hair long you have to be especially diligent about getting trims; damaged hair is particularly obvious when it's long.

your hair makeover

There is nothing as fun as having an expert makeover your hairstyle. In this chapter, we're going to give hair makeovers to several women of different ages, backgrounds, and hair types. I worked with Sacha, one of the greatest hairstylists I know and the only one who has cut my hair for the last seven years.

THE PERFECT BLOW OUT FOR FINE/STRAIGHT HAIR

Elizabeth was blessed with an amazing face and body but wanted to add volume to her baby-fine hair. Using the following steps, she achieved "movie-star" hair with very little effort.

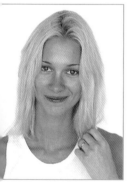

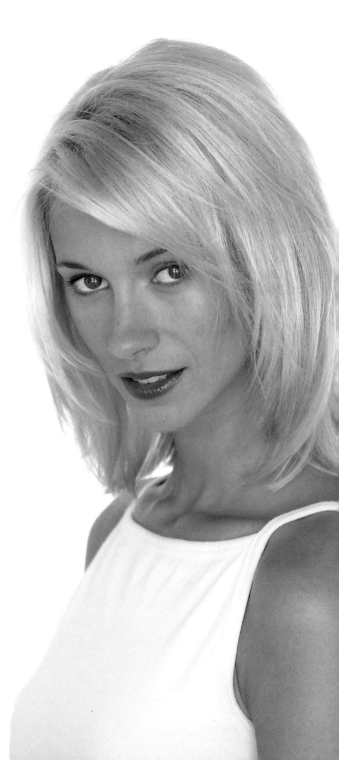

Wash and towel dry your hair to minimize dampness. Run a wide-toothed comb through your hair.

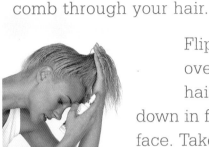

Flip your head over with the hair hanging down in front of your face. Take a thickening lotion or spray and cover the entire root area of your hair.

While leaning over, begin to blow-dry the roots first, lightly pulling the hair straight out with your fingers. This gives you volume from the root out.

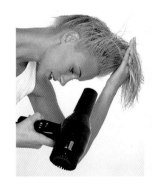

Flip your head back. Take large sections of your hair and wrap them around a medium-sized round brush, lightly pulling away from the head and slightly down as you blow-dry the hair on the brush. This gives you a smooth voluminous style. Taking sections from the front and top, do the same motion up and out with the brush.

If you like separation, take a tiny amount of molding mud between your index finger and thumb and apply to small pieces of your hair from the halfway mark to the end. Try and keep heavy products away from your roots so you don't weigh fine hair down.

CURLY HAIR, COARSE OR FINE

With this type of hair, loving it and leaving it alone is a smart way to start. Fighting it can turn you into a slave to straightening products and the weather. If your curly hair is also color-treated, then you also have to deal with breakage and split ends. With Jana, whose natural red hair is fabulous, we will demonstrate what I've learned over the last eleven years as the best way to care for thick, frizzy hair, leaving it soft and curly with no stiffness or frizz.

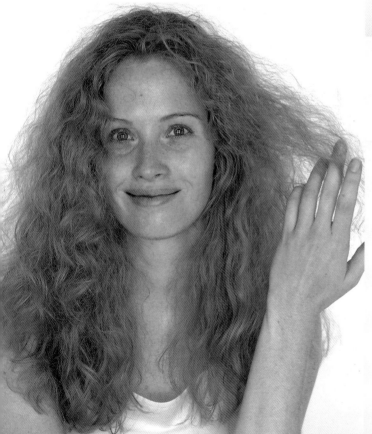

Shampoo with a light, nonstripping shampoo designed for dry and/or color-treated hair.

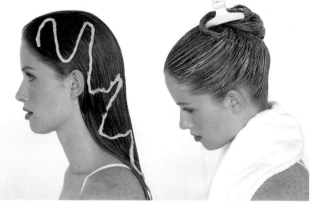

Apply a thick, deep-conditioning conditioner. If your hair is long, hold it back with a clip or a plastic cap so you can let the conditioner penetrate while you do your other shower duties.

After a few minutes, take your hair down. Comb through it gently with a wide-toothed comb or a pick, beginning at the ends. It takes a few minutes, but it's best to comb this type of hair in the shower while you have protective conditioners in it.

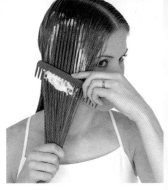

After you finish combing out your hair, put only the top of your head under the water. This way you can rinse the roots while leaving a little conditioner on the ends.

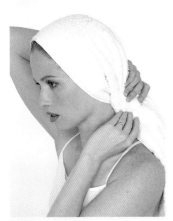

When you get out of the shower, wrap a towel gently around your head. You don't want to take all of the water out yet or the curling process will begin.

In the palm of your hand, mix together equal parts of a nice light gel that contains no silicone (see page 121) and a cream pomade or hairdressing that is also silicone-free. Without disturbing the hair too much, apply the mixture from the root to the ends of your hair. Make sure you cover your entire head so you don't have any frizzy hair poking through. You can use a little extra cream on the ends if you'd like.

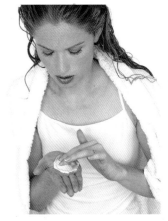

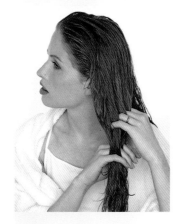

Now, with a small towel and with both hands, scrunch your hair from the tips up, gently guiding your curls into place, being care-

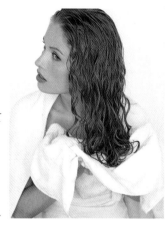

ful not to swing your hair or separate the curls too much. This process is key to a smooth, frizz-free drying process. I try to let my hair dry naturally as often as possible to avoid overheating; air drying also results in the nicest curls. If you're pressed for time or you can't leave the house with a wet head, use a dryer with a diffuser for a gentle drying process.

Once your hair is dry, use your fingers to gently separate the curls for a smooth curly look. Try to avoid running your fingers through your hair or it will begin to look frizzy. You can also use one of the lighter wax pomades on the roots around your hairline, to enhance the smoothness around your face. Give your head a gentle shake and you should see smooth, cascading curls without the frizz!

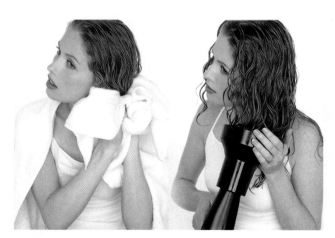

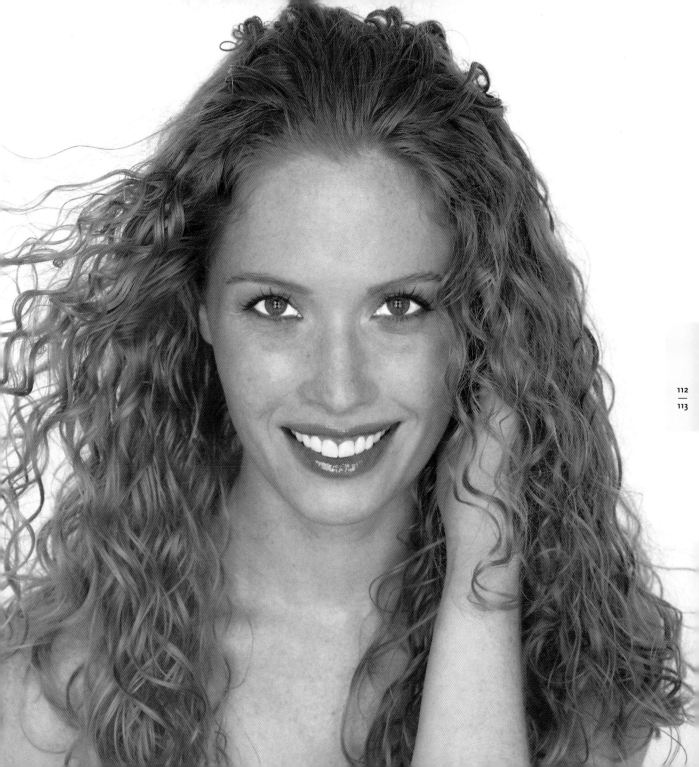

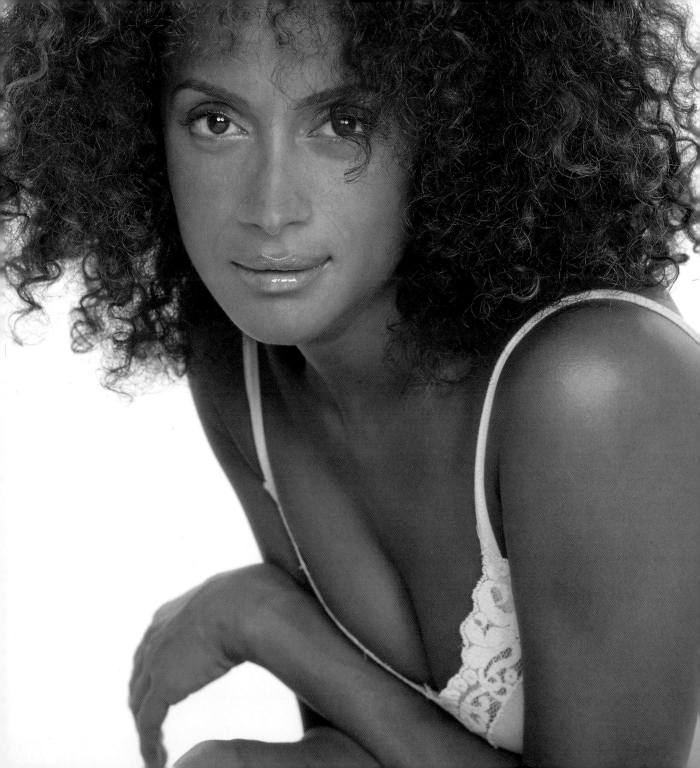

STRAIGHTENING EXTRA-CURLY HAIR— DAMAGE FREE!

Boy, is this something I know about. Unfortunately, I had to learn the hard way through years and years of different stylists burning my hair almost beyond repair. I eventually started requesting that clients tell me how they wanted my hair before I was booked, so I could straighten my own hair.

Using Marita as our model, I will demonstrate how to straighten very dry, relaxed or non-relaxed, curly or frizzy hair without damaging it. As you can see, Marita has wonderful natural curls. For a different look, she sometimes wants her hair to be straight without damaging it.

Straightening begins with the washing and conditioning process. If I'm going to straighten my hair, I wash my hair only with conditioner.

Towel dry the hair just enough to stop the drip. You'll want it to be very wet to prevent frizz from setting in. Some people swear by the straightening products available now and put them in before they start blow-drying, but I try to avoid using any products at this point. You can always add them to your hair after it's dry. For some people straightening products are a must; I would limit their use to a small quantity.

With a rat-tailed comb, separate your hair into sections, so you can concentrate on one section at a time without the others drying. Twist each one and hold it back with a clip.

Blow-dry your hair as you wrap it around a large round brush. The brush 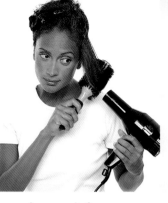 will seem slightly awkward for your hands at first but if you take up small sections of hair it will be easier. After you straighten your hair with the round brush, use a flat brush to "bump" any curl that the round brush may have missed.

As you finish each section, twist the hair and put it back up in a small bun while you work the remaining sections. This is important because it gives the hair a chance to cool without being exposed to the humidity caused by the blow-dryer on your wet hair. Otherwise you'll have to keep drying the sections over and over again.

When you've dried all of the sections and have clipped them all up again, let your hair cool for a few minutes. Then take all the sections down at the same time. Using the flat brush, simply dry your entire head at once. This will eliminate any bends that the clips may have left and give you a nice uniform look. If you want a more voluminous style you can use the round brush on the top section and dry it straight up, pulling away from your crown. If you want it to be "piecier" you can add some water-free pomade to the hair but make sure you keep it away from the root or you'll make that area dirty.

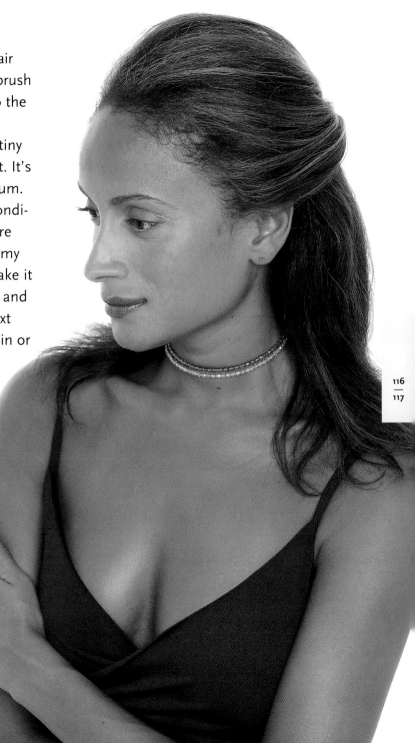

Ideally you should be able to keep your hair straight for three or four days. At night I brush it out to distribute the natural sebum to the ends, and then I wrap it up. If you feel that your hair is very dry you can add a tiny amount of jojoba oil to the ends at night. It's the closest oil in nature to our own sebum.

It's important to keep your hair conditioned after straightening. The day before I'm ready to wash my hair again, I coat my hair with just enough shea butter to make it pliable. Then I put it in braids or a bun and keep it up all day and overnight. The next day I wash it and either straighten it again or leave it curly.

FIVE-MINUTE HAIR

Christie is a beautiful, athletic, new mom.
She is not a primper, and only spends about
five minutes on her hair. So we gave her a
cut that will look great with only five minutes
of styling. She has a long, narrow face with
fine features. This cut also has the advantage
of shaping the hair around the face to highlight her beautiful face and cheekbones.

The next is Nanou: a wonderful woman
from France who takes her body and mind
very seriously. She runs six miles a day and
has completed several marathons. She needs
easy, sophisticated hair that she can change
for whatever country or event she's going to.
We gave her a great, short cut that can easily
be styled for either a sporty, casual look or
an elegant look for the evening. By thinning
out her top-heavy hairstyle, we helped enhance
her great features.

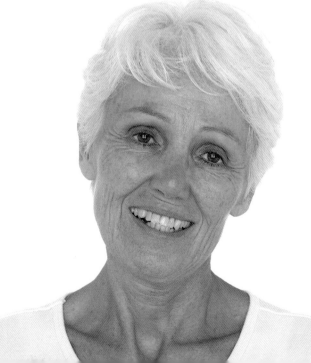

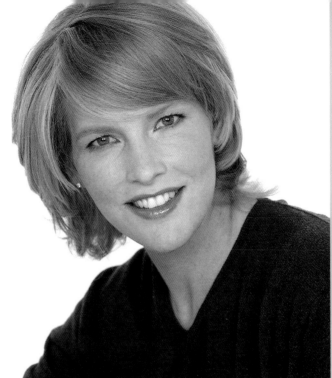

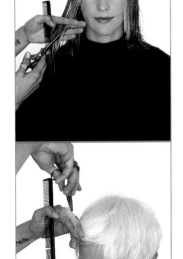

hot tip

THE ONLY THING WORSE
THAN A BAD HAIR DAY
IS A BAD HAIRCUT.
THEN EVERY DAY IS A
BAD HAIR DAY UNTIL IT
GROWS OUT. WHEN
THIS HAPPENS, I RECOM-
MEND YOU CUT A CLEAN,
STRAIGHT LINE, AS
SHORT AS YOU CAN
STAND. KEEP IT AT THAT
LENGTH UNTIL THE TOP
LAYERS CATCH UP
TO THE BOTTOM. YOU
WILL END UP WITH
A BLUNT CUT THAT CAN
BE MADE INTO MANY
DIFFERENT STYLES.

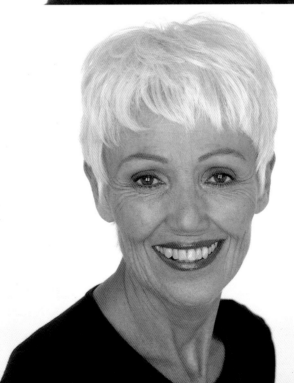

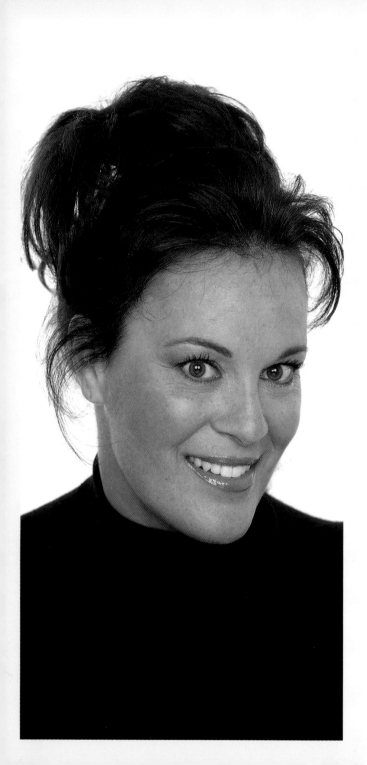

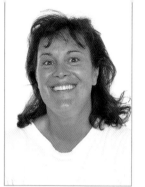

DON'T HIDE BEHIND YOUR HAIR

My sister Beth is a beautiful woman with gorgeous brown hair. She always wears her hair down to cover her full face. I wanted to show you how a little makeup and an easy up-style can make your face look dramatically slimmer. I didn't do any contouring with makeup, I just changed the shape of her hair to show her long neck and emphasize her fabulous eyes. Keeping the softness with the tendrils around the face makes her look sleek, yet soft.

Coloring

I have had the pleasure of having one of the world's great colorists make my dark ash blond hair look naturally beautiful and sunlit. I can understand the old saying that you can replace a husband easier than a great colorist. If you can afford having a professional color your hair, I would highly recommend it, at least for the first time. Pay attention and ask questions. If you go repeatedly to the same colorist, he or she might even give you your formula—if you ask nicely.

I am also a seasoned professional when it comes to coloring my own hair. I have even had to color my hair in foreign countries without being able to read what's on the carton. The key to finding the right color is scrutinizing your natural color. Look in the mirror. Is it an ash or a red tone? Based on that you will be able to decide where to go from there. Just remember that the more you change from your natural color the more maintenance your hair will need.

I color my hair in two steps. First I do what's called a "single process," applying one color from the root to the tip. Whether the purpose is to lighten or darken, the root line will always be visible with a single process. Then I do highlights, which are very common today. Cream or powder bleach is either painted on or applied with a fine comb and tin foil to completely strip the color from the hair. Because you are changing only selected hairs, highlighting is less noticeable and requires less maintenance.

SILICONE WARNING

SEVERAL YEARS AGO, MANUFACTURERS BEGAN TO ADD SILICONE, A DERIVATIVE OF SAND, TO HAIR PRODUCTS. AT FIRST I WAS A TOTAL JUNKIE. I COATED MY HAIR WITH SILICONE AND HAIR GEL AND EITHER BLOW-DRIED IT OR LET IT DRY CURLY. AFTER SEVERAL MONTHS OF THIS, MY STYLIST AND I STARTED TO SEE A MASS OF BREAKAGE ON MY HAIR. NEITHER OF US COULD FIGURE IT OUT. WITH A LITTLE INVESTIGATION WE DISCOVERED THAT THE SILICONE WAS DESTROYING MY HAIR. SILICONE IS SUPPOSED TO BENEFIT YOUR HAIR BY COATING AND SEALING THE HAIR SHAFT AND CUTICLE SO THAT NO MOISTURE CAN PENETRATE IT. BUT BECAUSE MY HAIR IS COARSE, CURLY, DRY, AND COLOR-TREATED, IT NEEDS CONSTANT MOISTURE RENEWAL. WITHOUT MOISTURE, MY HAIR WAS BREAKING OFF. SILICONE MIGHT NOT BE A PROBLEM FOR YOU IF YOU HAVE SHORT HAIR THAT GETS CUT OFTEN, BUT SINCE I BEGAN TO LIMIT MY USE OF IT TO IMPORTANT JOBS ONLY, MY HAIR HAS CONTINUED TO GROW AND FLOURISH. SILICONE GOES BY MANY NAMES, ONE BEING DIMETHICONE. IF WHEN LOOKING AT PRODUCTS YOU SEE ANY CHEMICAL NAME THAT ENDS WITH CONE IT'S USUALLY A DERIVATIVE OF SILICONE.

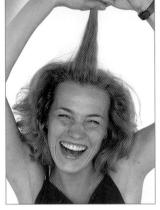

COLOR CORRECTING

If you are unhappy with the color of your hair there are some very easy adjustments you can make to correct it. Within the first forty-eight hours you can wash repeatedly with a strong color-stripping shampoo. This will dramatically lighten newly colored hair.

If your hair is overhighlighted and brassy, it's easy to fix. Choose a semipermanent hair color a few shades lighter than your own. With a paintbrush or a toothbrush, apply what are called "low-lights" to your hair. By carefully painting streaks of a darker color, you break up that solid, flat appearance. What you don't want is one color throughout your entire head (look at a child's hair—it has many different colors in it). Creating low-lights is not difficult, but it takes patience and the ability to paint in a semistraight line. Just remember that overprocessed hair is incredibly porous, so whatever color you put on will soak into the hair follicle quickly. You'll have to watch carefully to make sure your hair doesn't pick up too much of the dark color.

Sophie is a professional equestrian who has colored her hair one too many times and would like to have an at-home permanent coloring to bring her hair back to its natural shade. We did a single-process semipermanent color on Sophie, using her eyebrows and body hair color as a guide.

Choose a semipermanent color because overprocessed hair is very porous. A rinse will wash out too quickly. Using petroleum jelly or a thick cream conditioner, go around your hairline to protect your skin from being dyed. Follow the instructions on the package very carefully.

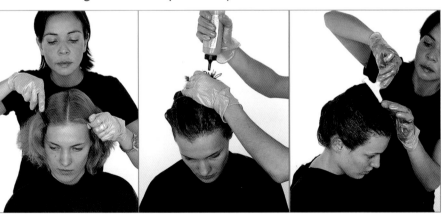

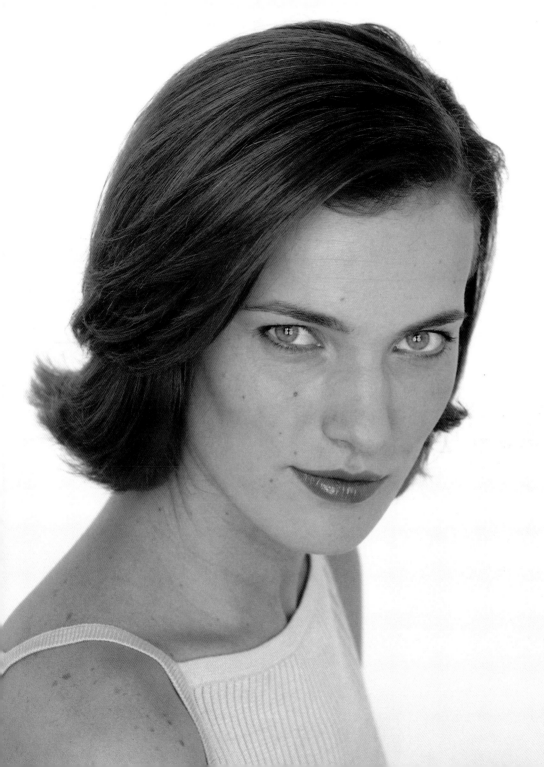

To extend the life of your color, wait as long as you can after coloring to wash it. It takes time for the color to adhere completely to the follicle. If hair is washed within the first forty-eight hours of coloring, up to sixty percent of the color could wash out. When you do wash your hair, use a light shampoo designed for color-treated hair.

hair accessories

One of the great things about modeling is seeing what others would do to give you a new look. It's amazing what accessories can do to add spice to an outfit or hairstyle. Most women either never do anything with their hair or they do too much. To demonstrate how to create four different looks with accessories, we used Audra, a sixteen-year-old who usually leaves her hair down. These easy, affordable options are great for women of all ages. The accessories might inspire you to be creative with your hair no matter what your busy schedule dictates.

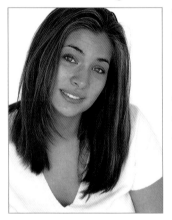

Twisting the hair for the beach or athletics. This is an easy alternative to the ponytail. Take a small section from the front of your hair, twist it, and clip it in the back. Add more twists and add new clips as they get full. When you've twisted all the hair on top from ear to ear, gather all the hair and put it in a ponytail holder, wrapping it tightly so the twists don't come loose. You can spray it with a little hair spray if you have fly-away hairs.

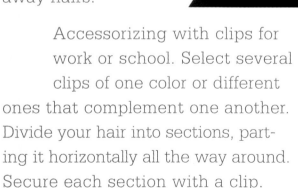

Accessorizing with clips for work or school. Select several clips of one color or different ones that complement one another. Divide your hair into sections, parting it horizontally all the way around. Secure each section with a clip.

You can put the clips in a straight or jagged line, covering your entire head. Be creative. You can 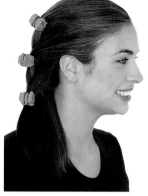 also tie ribbons around your clips, securing them with glue, to transform plain clips into beautiful accessories.

Accessorizing with flex combs for an evening out. Flex combs are inexpensive and easy to find, either plain or with beads or ribbons on them. Starting at the front of your hairline, slip the combs toward the back of your head. The first one should end at the top of the head. Keep adding combs until you have the look you want. If you have fine hair, you may have to tease it a little so that the combs will stay in.

Special-occasion hair. This is a variation on the last style but it uses many different head bands, clips, and flex combs. Have the look in mind before you start adding accessories to your hair. Make sure your hair is perfectly combed and secure. This style takes about two minutes to do but will last for a whole night of dancing. Try to ease up on other jewelry and accessories when you wear your hair like this so you don't look like you're wearing everything you own.

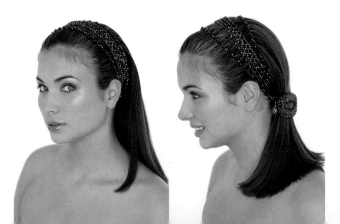

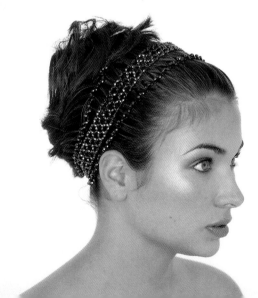

innovations
in hair

At a certain point in a woman's life she may experience hair loss due to changes in hormones, pregnancy, stress, age, etc. But fortunately, just as with everything in our lives, the hair market has grown by leaps and bounds. You can now use extensions and hairpieces to make your everyday hair fuller or more glamorous.

HAIR EXTENSIONS

Hair extensions are a great way to transform thin or short hair into long, voluminous locks. My recommendation is that you seek a professional consultation for hair extensions if you want to keep them in for more than a day. The permanent way to extend your hair is through weaving or sewing the hair extension into your existing hair. There is also a gluing method that is quick and easy.

We used Caroline to illustrate a beautiful full-sewn weave. She has a short bob and wanted long hair. This weave, which would take only a few hours to do, will stay intact for three to four months. Every couple of weeks she returns to the professional to get the roots tightened, because as your hair grows the length will pull the thread loose. Remember that the sewn weaves will be costly. The average cost of a real hair weave is $500 to $1,000.

HAIRPIECES

The easiest way to enhance your hair is to attach a hairpiece yourself. You can buy clip or comb tufts for around $50. They are similar to old-fashioned hairpieces but instead of being overly coifed they are now simple hair extensions with clips or combs sewn to the base. You simply part your hair, attach the clip underneath, and then fold your hair over so you can't see the top. You may need to tease the base of the hair where you are attaching the clip if you have thin hair; this will help keep the clip in much longer.

Natural hairpieces usually come in one length: medium to long. You can cut them to the length you want or bring them to a stylist. Hairpieces are available in a variety of colors, but you can dye them yourself or take them to a colorist.

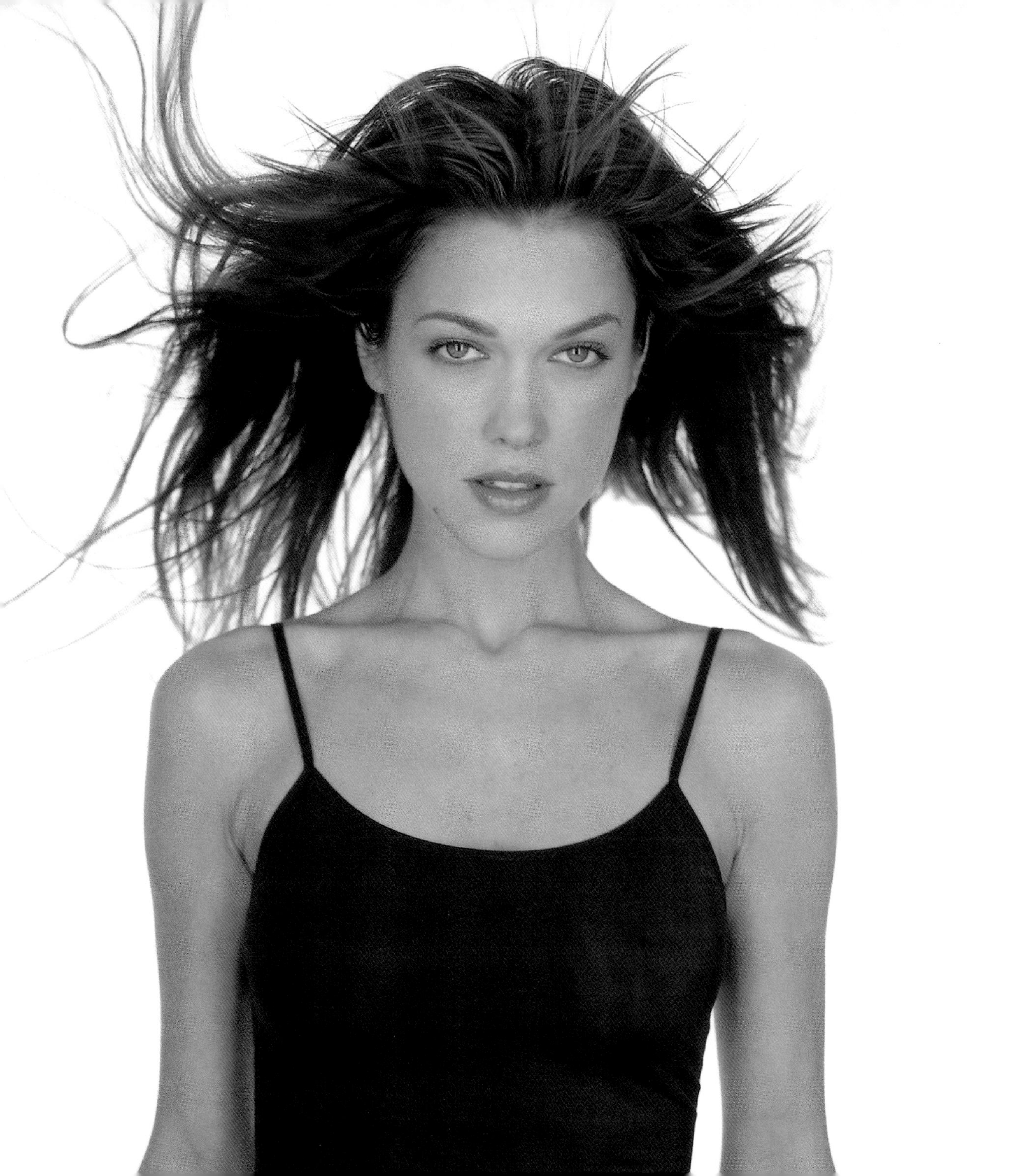

your nails

A model's hands and nails must be beautiful. Luckily, doing your own manicure is easy and fun. A weekly manicure should be part of your beauty routine, not an occasional indulgence. If I don't have time to get a professional manicure, I will do my own using my little manicure kit. Because I travel so much and can't bring my manicurist on trips with me, over the years I have experimented with every brand and type of nail product imaginable. I have used the tea bag mending kit in England and I've done my nails in every part of the world. When I get to my hotel I run a hot bubble bath, take off all my nail polish, and soak. What I'm really soaking are my hands and feet.

In this chapter, I'll show you how easy it is to do your own manicure and pedicure and make it look like the work of a professional.

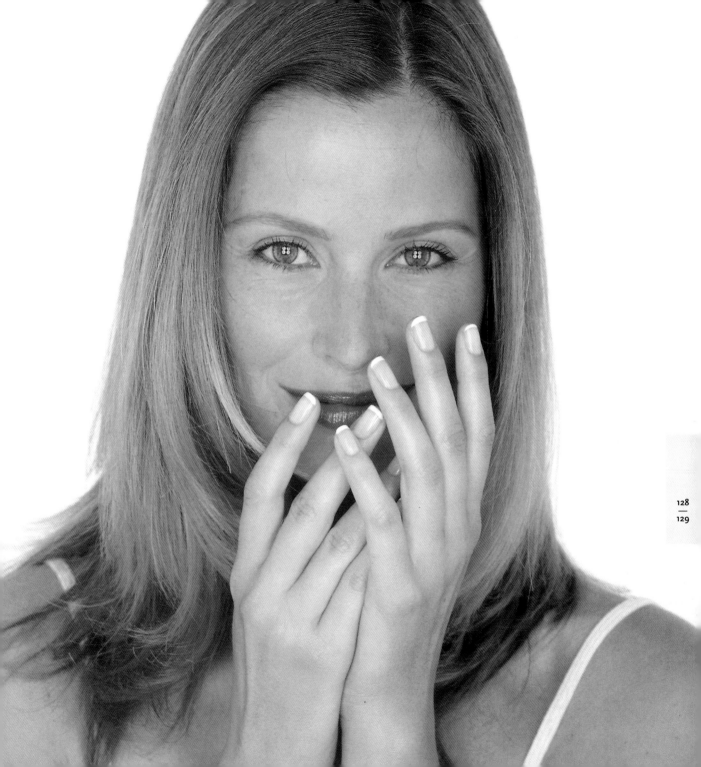

For most catalogs, a model's nails are expected to be a natural pink or a soft color. Personally I like a French manicure with an off-white tip, although I do love all the great new colors that are out now. Feel free to try different colors and combinations—remember that nail polish can be easily removed. If you end up with something you don't like, you can take it right off. I love it when I see a woman with fun colors. It shows me she's not afraid to play with her look.

essential nail care products

1 Acetone-free polish remover. For travel, the remover pads that are individually wrapped are best for easy packing.

2 Cotton pads if you can't find the individually wrapped pads.

3 An all-purpose foam nail file or a sapphire nail file for delicate or weak nails.

4 A round buffer file or block for buffing rough edges after filing.

5 A cream- or oil-based cuticle remover.

6 A plastic stick or several orangewood sticks for pushing back your cuticles.

7 A sharp, pointed pair of scissors or a metal cuticle remover.

8 A stiff-haired brush to help remove dead skin around cuticles and clean under nails.

9 A base coat that has a strengthener or one that can be used as a top coat as well.

10 An off-white opaque color for your French manicure tip.

11 A pink or beige (depending on your skin color and preference) sheer second coat for over the white tip.

12 Mending paper or silk, or a tea bag.

13 Nail mending glue suitable for sensitive skin.

14 Mending powder for extra strength.

15 Manicure clean-up stick.

16 Quick-dry spray.

THE HOME MANICURE

Clean your nail polish off with the remover pads or remove with cotton pads.

Fill a small bowl with soapy water or a cuticle-soaking product. Soak your nails for several minutes and dry them off.

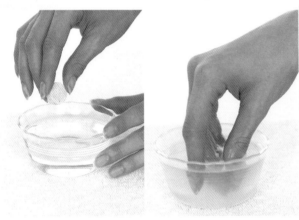

Carefully file your nails with the appropriate file, making sure that you file in one direction. Filing back and forth tears up the ends of your nails and makes them rough around the edges. Depending on the shape and length of your fingers, determine how long you want your nails. The most attractive length for my nails is just slightly longer than my finger-

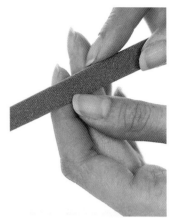

tips. After you decide whether you want a square tip or a round tip, you can follow that guide for each nail. Remember to turn your hand around to check that the nail is even when it's peeking over the top of your finger.

With the buffer square, gently file the top and outside edge of your nail to make sure that the edges are nice and smooth. Filing up and under the nail is good for eliminating any loose edges.

Next, take the cuticle oil or cream and spread a dab on each nail of your left hand then turn your hand over and put a dab on the pad of each finger so you can then spread the cream on your other hand. Once you've spread the cream over your fingers, knead it around your cuticles—getting it under the nail bed will prevent or alleviate hangnails. Allow your skin to absorb it for about five minutes.

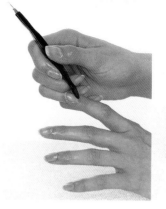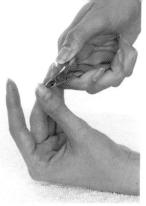

bed and if you cut them you could prevent future growth or cause infections; if you damage your cuticles you are causing damage to the new growth. When you use a cuticle cutter or scissors make sure that you only cut where you have hangnails or loose skin around the fingernail.

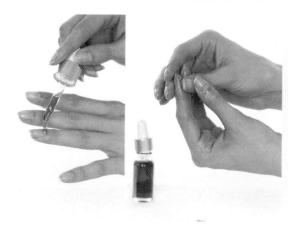

Take the cuticle stick and gently push your cuticles back. Be careful, because your cuticles are there to protect your nail

After you trim away the dead skin, gently scrub with the brush and tepid water in a circular motion to remove any remaining dead skin. Your nails should feel squeaky clean now. If after you wash your hands you see little pieces of nail that didn't get filed, you can use the buffer to file them off.

8 Apply a thin layer of base coat.

9 Wait about two minutes and apply the light-pink coat.

10 Again wait a few minutes. If you need French tip guides you can put them on the tips of your nails now. You will probably need to use these guides the first couple of times you do this manicure.

11 With the opaque off-white color, paint the tips, following the lines around the tip guides. Again, allow the polish a few minutes to dry. If you can get a nice thick line with one swipe, that's ideal. I think two coats of the white tip looks too thick, and it takes forever to dry.

12 Now apply one coat of the pink or beige sheer polish, in as thin and sheer a layer as possible.

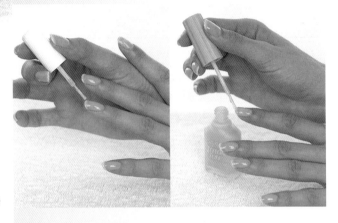

13 After your color is done you should wait another three to four minutes and then apply the top coat sealer (or dual base/top coat) to your nails. A top coat is very important to add life and longevity to your nail enamel. I add another coat later in the week for additional protection.

If you make any mistakes you can use the "mistake pen"—a pen with nail polish remover on its tip—to clean things up. If you do your nails in the evening and take a shower after they dry, you can usually clean up your nails in the shower, as the steam and heat help remove the polish from your skin. But remember that water tends to soften your nails and shorten the life of a manicure. I always use gloves while housecleaning.

If you have wrapped nails or acrylic nails there are many products on the market now that are specifically designed to mend or "fill" your artificial nails. I love having my nails wrapped but it's expensive and you must keep it up or you'll end up with weaker nails than you started with.

I regularly use a cuticle-softening stick, an all-natural glide-on stick that I apply to my nails and hands and then to my elbows right before bed. I don't like to cover my hands with cotton gloves while I sleep, so this is the next best thing. If you do this every night as part of your bedtime routine I promise you will have soft and beautiful fingers, hands, and elbows.

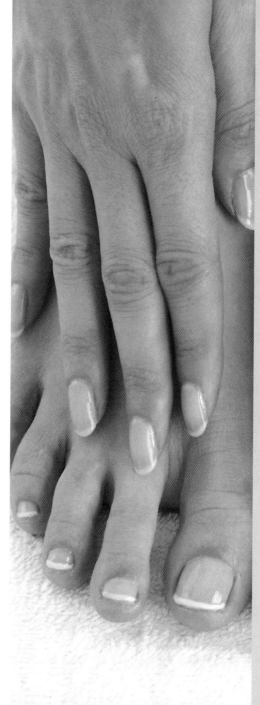

hot tip

IF YOU DON'T HAVE POLISH REMOVER, YOU CAN USE YOUR TOP COAT POLISH INSTEAD. BRUSH A GENEROUS AMOUNT ON YOUR SKIN AND NAIL AND WIPE OFF WITH A PAPER NAPKIN.

FIXING A BROKEN NAIL
Fixing a broken nail is as easy as having a cup of tea.

Carefully unfold a new tea bag (before it has been soaked in boiling water) and pour out all the tea.

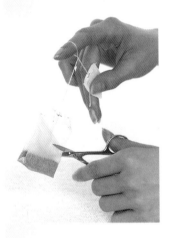 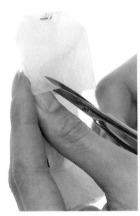

Using the fingernail bed as a guide, cut a patch of the tea-bag paper a little bigger than the actual break or rip in your nail. Make sure your nail is clean and unpolished; this will make the fabric adhere better.

Place the paper on the break and soak it with nail glue (or super glue) until the paper becomes transparent.

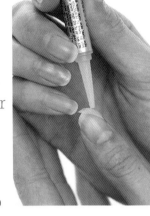

Be careful not to touch it, because it will be very sticky. Let it dry for a moment and then add another coat of glue. You can also add a nail powder to strengthen the nail further.

After it is completely dry, use a semi-coarse file and file the glue until it is smooth. A coat of clear polish will seal it further and then you can use any nail color you wish.

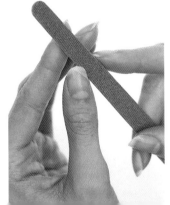

THE EASY PEDICURE

I had my first pedicure ten years ago with my friend Marita. I couldn't believe my feet were in such bad shape. I have big feet (size 11—what a drag). But after seeing how much the pedicure improved my feet, I vowed that while I couldn't change the size of my feet at least I would make sure that they were beautiful. I have been either having them professionally done or have maintained them myself once a week ever since.

I gave my mother her first pedicure and have enjoyed doing them for my grandmother as well. If I can teach Virginia how to do this herself, anyone can do it!

I'm sure you're thinking an easy pedicure is a contradiction but I assure you that this will be fast and easy. All you have to do is prepare yourself and you can do your own pedicure with very little time and energy. You can do it with the same tools as your manicure; if you're in a hurry you can substitute a shower or bath for a bowl of water for soaking your feet.

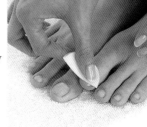

Remove any preexisting nail polish.

Then paint cuticle remover lotion liberally all over your toenails right before you jump in the shower or tub.

A nice long soaking bath will make your pedicure easier, but a five- to ten-minute shower will do the job.

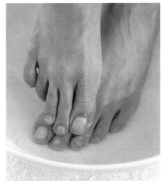

After your shower, bath, or soak, apply another coat of cuticle remover to your toes, and using a toenail clipper, cut straight across your toenails, making sure you

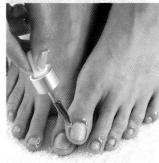

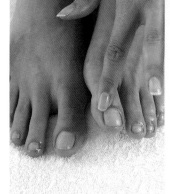

don't cut them too short (this will cause your skin to grow over the top of your toe, which can be painful).

5 File the nails straight across, moving the file in the same direction. Special toenail files can be purchased at any drugstore and make filing easy and fast.

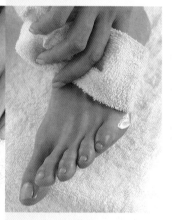

6 With your orangewood cuticle stick, push your cuticles back all around your toes. You should find that the shower helped to soften

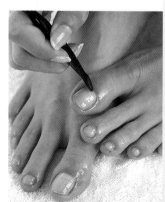

your cuticles. If you have any hang-skin (I never understood why they call it a hangnail when it's really loose skin bits), snip it off.

7 Spray some water over your toes, rub them gently with a scrub brush to get rid of any dead skin, and then wipe them with a towel. I like to step back into the tub and give my feet and nails a good scrub, but it's up to you.

8 With lotion and a pumice stone, scrub all over your feet, concentrating on the heel and any corns on the sides (I am forever stuffing

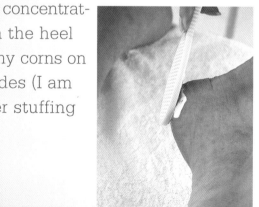

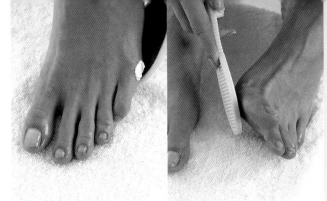

too much attention to themselves, but colors can be fun, too. Remember that if you do a French pedicure you have to allow at least four hours before you put closed-toe shoes on.

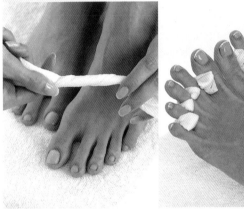

my size-11 feet into size-9 shoes so I've suffered the consequences). Scrub the corns as much as you can, then rinse again and pat dry with a towel.

9 Now that the initial cleaning and maintenance are done you can either stop and just leave your feet bare or you can add polish. As with my fingernails I prefer a French pedicure and apply it the same way as I do my fingernails. I find that my feet always look clean and pretty without drawing

Maintaining your hands and feet should be fun and rewarding. The best thing I can tell you is that the time and energy you spend on them you get back tenfold in compliments. I get compliments on my feet almost every time I wear open-toed shoes. When I say, "not bad for a size eleven," the person usually can't believe they're so big.

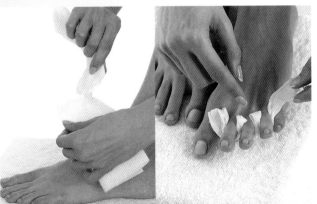

your
lifestyle

A true makeover should really incorporate changes beyond your skin, makeup, hair, and nails. It should include changes to your lifestyle, such as wearing clothes that make you feel confident, beginning a new exercise regimen, improving your eating habits, and developing a healthy attitude. It should also include improving your mind. I am an avid reader of books on many different topics, from suspense thrillers to self-help and spirituality. But you might also want to take a course, pick up a hobby, or cultivate new interests. The important thing is that you always use your mind and body, which will help enrich your lifestyle. This may sound daunting, but if you start with small steps, you'll be amazed by how quickly you begin to see improvements on the outside, and feel them on the inside.

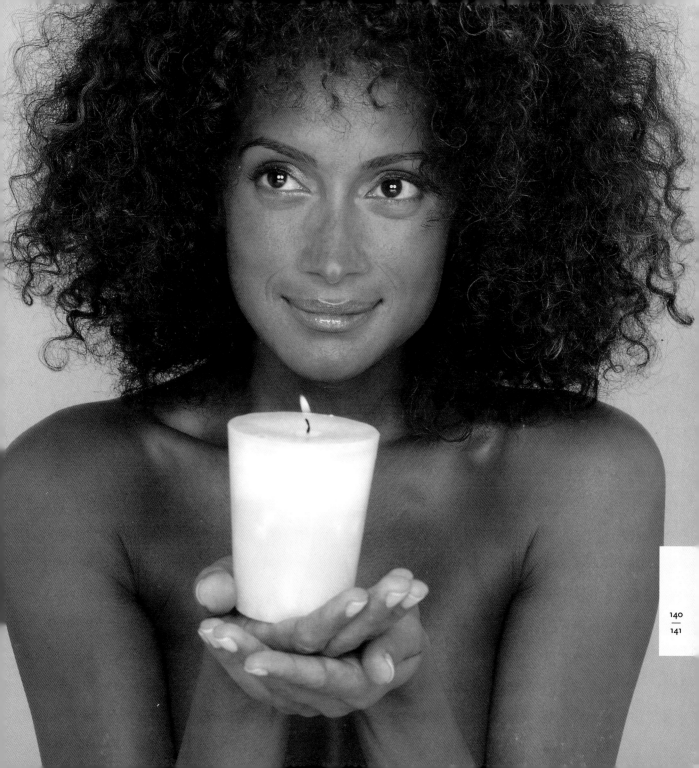

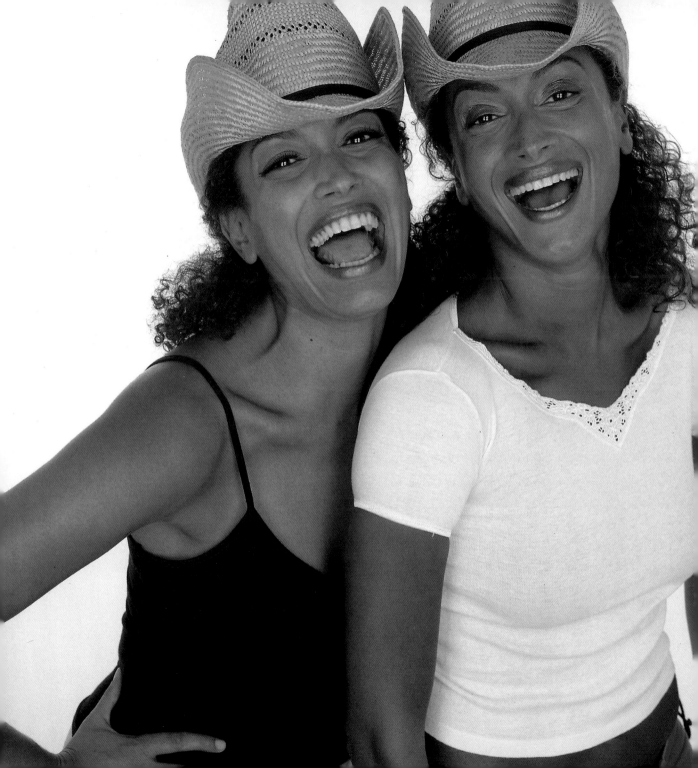

clothing and fashion

Trying on new clothing every day is one of the most fabulous things about being a model. (It is also an easy way to completely make yourself over.) The key is seeing what the designers are showing and knowing how to make it work for us. There are some things that a woman should definitely splurge on and others that you can find at a discount or even in vintage clothing shops.

Working with your own personal style and knowing your body type is where you begin. I end up being a stylist to my family and many of my friends because I've worn every type of clothing and fabric imaginable. I am very picky when it comes to fabrics and cuts. When you're trying to define your personal style it's easiest to simply plagiarize one or many other people's styles. I'm always checking out magazines and catalogs, looking at what I think might be a successful look for me. I then try to find something like it in vintage clothing stores before I buy an expensive piece—almost everything has been done before. Every year in the fashion industry they are saying that the eighties are like the sixties or the nineties are like the seventies. So I'm always popping by the local thrift store wherever I travel; it's fun to find that one special piece that brings your whole outfit together. I also keep a list of the basic wardrobe pieces that I need. For instance, I'm always looking for that perfect long black winter coat. I have it written in my calendar so it's always in the back of my mind.

Another great idea is to pick out your favorite colors and buy a few inexpensive tops in those colors. Then when you wear the tops, listen to what others say about you so you can be aware of what colors look good on you. I love blue and red. Every time I wear a certain top I always feel like my skin looks good and people compliment my eyes. Now that I know that I like the color and that others seem to think I look good in it, I can keep on the lookout for more expensive high-quality pieces to include in my permanent wardrobe. This way you don't have a closet full of clothes that you don't love, and you can weed out the not-so-great colors, replacing them with your better colors without breaking the bank.

The media constantly bombards us with what models and celebrities are wearing. The average woman in America is 5'5" and a size 14. In this chapter I will show all women how they can dress beautifully no matter what their size, shape, or style may be. Borrowing from men's fashions and mixing them with vintage or items from the large size selection is a great way to expand your choices while remaining comfortable. Let's just say, "No more muumuus!"

Your Body Shape

I know we've heard a million times that women come in four shapes: the apple, pear, figure 8, or the straight up and down. Well, I believe we're all variations of those four themes. I've always thought that at the beginning of a clothing catalog there should be a front- and side-view picture of each model wearing a leotard and tights, so you could go through the catalog and find what looks best on the model with the figure closest to your own. It's even more difficult to shop from a catalog knowing that what you're seeing in a picture is nothing close to what it looked like before pinning and fittings began.

The best way to find the right style and cut for you is to go to a large department store, where you can try lots of looks on in one place and find what you like. You don't have to buy at those prices but at least you can determine that, say, three-quarter-length sleeves make your arms look trim and slender. Then when you find a top on sale with three-quarter-length sleeves you can snatch it up. This is how you build a wardrobe. Most of my friends and family hate to shop. I love not only shopping for myself but also for all of the people in my life—and most of my non-shopping friends have learned over the years to trust my judgment. I also try to push the envelope with both my looks and those of my friends. I like to change my style all the time. For me, clothes are like playing dress-up every day of my life!

Pear-Shaped Women

Pear-shaped women have an especially varied selection of clothes to choose from right now. The boot-cut pant for example, is very popular and easy to find. The slightly wider ankle balances a heavy thigh or hip so your legs look thinner and longer. Add a three-quarter-length fitted jacket and a nice mid-heel boot and you have a wonderful, voluptuous silhouette.

Apple Girls

No, you don't look like an apple, but you carry most of your weight around your middle and you have beautiful legs. (I'm a pear wishing

I had the legs of an apple girl!) The biggest mistake you can make is wearing long tent dresses or anything that covers those great gams. If your arms are heavy or make you uncomfortable then a three-quarter-length sleeve is perfect for you. You get the lengthening effect without always having to wear long sleeves.

As an apple girl, you also have a nice chest, so V-necks and good bras should be staples in your wardrobe. Be on the lookout for camisoles to wear under fitted blazers, and remember that blazers with a small but shapely shoulder pad can make your waist look smaller. But I stress the word small when I speak of shoulder pads. You can look like a football player in no time if the shoulder pads are too large—they tend to make your neck disappear. So be conscious of your entire silhouette. You want to look longer, leaner, and evenly distributed. Heels are usually good for lengthening a torso: any heels with a slight incline will make you taller and subsequently, if your posture is correct, help bring your shoulders back. If you are busty be very mindful of your posture. Nothing adds weight more than slouching shoulders.

Figure 8
You have the best of both worlds: an ample bust, a small waist, and hips. You're easy to shop for as long as you love your shape. I have friends who don't love being voluptuous, and I don't get it. It's the best part of being a woman. Show it off! Lycra should be your friend! Keeping good taste in mind while having fun with all different styles of clothing is a pleasure. Fitted clothing usually looks good on you because the smaller waist balances the shoulders and hips. I recommend the boot-cut pant again, for the simple reason that it shows off the hip while keeping a long leg. The fashion world is your oyster—you have so many choices.

Straight Up and Down (Boy Shaped)
You, too, can wear most clothing styles. Preference and fit are entirely individual matters, but there's more out there for your type than for the others. The only recommendation I have is to emphasize your waist. Clothes that make it look like you have some curves will make you feel sexier. I'd try some of the new V-shaped low-cut pants, because the V helps draw the line down so your waist looks smaller than your hips. Of course you can't go show up at the office with these

pants, but for evenings they can be very cute. Anything that is fitted in the waist will do the job as well. There are many shirts that are fitted like men's shirts with a little Lycra to make your waist shapely. Belts are good for that, too.

LOCATION, LOCATION, LOCATION
Knowing where to find the greatest clothes is another thing you pick up as a model. Not every model has clothing given to them by designers. If you live in a metropolitan area you can call different clothing lines and ask them where and when their sample sales are on. These are held twice a year. If you don't live in a big city, then try the myriad outlets that have popped up in the last few years. I like Neiman Marcus Last Call and Off Fifth (from Saks Fifth Avenue).

The key to sample and outlet shopping is going through your closet at least once a year. If you haven't worn it in a year you probably won't, so give it to someone else or to a charity. Then start making outfits. Pull out your favorite pants and tops and decide which one new piece could make them new or trendy. Keep a list and take it with you when you shop. Remember: If you don't need it, it doesn't matter if you got it cheap!

exercise and nutrition

Maintaining your figure is a challenge for most women, but when your body is your resume it is doubly important. Finding balance between what your body's set point is and what you want it to look like is not an easy task. I recommend a combination of diet and exercise. Muscle burns more calories by just existing than fat does. Combining a cardio/fat-burning regime with weight training is ideal. I try to do as many different exercises as I can each week. The more you keep your body guessing, the less chance your body has to get used to an exercise and the less chance you have for getting bored with your routine. __Exercise in the present__. Release any memories about what your body used to look like or what your fitness level was in the past. This helps you maintain your focus and stay in the "here and now" of your routines.

Nutrition is also multifaceted. I try to listen to my body and give it what it craves. I try to maintain moderation with regard to fats and sugars, but I don't live in a bubble. If I'm craving chocolate, I allow myself to indulge.

I try to work out as soon as possible after that, but I don't beat myself up over it. I take supplements, especially when I'm traveling a lot. They keep you steady in nutrients when you aren't eating correctly. There are many excellent books on supplements and herbal-remedies that can enhance your health and well-being. I believe in preventative health maintenance, which means that I try to avoid the carcinogens that could harm my long-term health and add the nutrients that I know will keep my immune system strong and my body clean. I use all of the resources available to me: homeopathy, herbs, chiropractic, nutritional supplements, organic food, exercise therapy, dental hygiene, and colon care. This doesn't mean that I don't have regular checkups with my medical doctors, just that I use all forms of medicine available to me.

Remember to check with your doctor before embarking on a new fitness routine. I know everyone says this, but it really is important. Think of it in terms of preventive health maintenance and not a checkup.

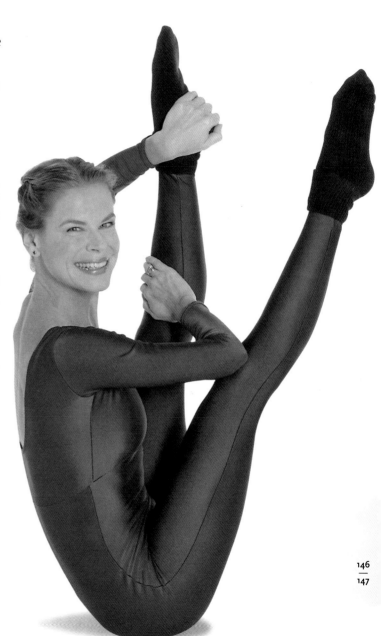

THE COMPLETE MAKEOVER

A long-term diet and exercise routine will show results in only a few weeks, but, with maintenance, it can make a drastic change. I will show you simple routines and combinations of exercises that can shape your body while you shed fat. A boot-camp–style routine is a fun two-week total body program; it gets you into the exercise mood.

There are many different theories on what you need to have a fit body. You'll get many different answers to the questions you ask. I base my fitness routine on what I know I will stick to, execution time, and results. I always do "preventive" exercises. This means that if bad knees are in your family, then you shouldn't do exercises that are stressful to your knees.

Take stock of your true fitness level. Think about what hurts when you wake up in the morning. Think about possible hereditary ailments—you may not have them now but if you abuse your body they may turn up later.

Figure out what you love to do. Do you like jogging? I know that there is a lot of research concluding that jogging can be tough on the body, but I have been jogging for almost my entire life. I wasn't born with a speedy metabolism, and I must exercise regularly (and jogging is a big part of my routine) in order to be able to eat with some enjoyment. If you loathe jogging, or it is simply too painful for you, then you must find another exercise that increases your heart rate to 65 to 85% of your maximum.

Compute your target heart rate. Subtract your age from 220. Take between 65% to 85% of that number. Let say you're 40. 220 minus 40 is 180. 65% of 180 is 117. That is your low target. 85% of 180 is 153. That would be your highest target. Now you must take into account what your current fitness level is. If you haven't lifted a finger in ten years then you should begin exercising in the low target range, or around 117 to 120. If you move your body at this range for at least 15 minutes you will begin burning fat. Now, if you are lifting weights, using resistance training, and keeping your heart rate at that level you are not only burning fat but you are also tearing down muscle fibers. They keep repairing for at least 24 hours, which means that our bodies have to work overtime—burning calories and building muscle mass.

Make an appointment with yourself. Okay I know we're all very busy. I have a hard time making the time to call my family regularly let alone the time to plan a workout, but that's exactly what you have to do. I plan my workouts just like appointments or meetings. If you enjoy going to exercise classes, planning is a little easier, because they are usually on set schedules. If you are a "lone" exerciser then you have to plan it or make it something you do without even thinking.

On my cardio days I jog first thing in the morning or I will find 50 reasons why I can't. I wake up, put my sneakers on, and go out the door before I have a chance to second-guess my schedule. On the days that I have a class or do weight training, I make an appointment in my calendar. You should give your muscles a day off between workouts or alternate muscle groups, so plan accordingly.

Choose your weapon. Exercise is supposed to be fun, but if you're like me, and love only the last thirty seconds of a workout because you know it's about to be over, then read on. One of my favorite classes is called the Lotte Berk Method. Currently available on the East Coast of the United States, it's a combination of strengthening and stretching exercises based on the disciplines of ballet, modern dance, yoga, and orthopedic back exercises. You don't need any dance training or background to do this. It is a non-impact class that increases your heart rate. The only drawback is that you must attend classes. They have books but they don't have a video-tape, and because the instructors are so highly trained and consistently retrained, they will not let the practice go to all gyms. I agree with them completely, but I do wish every person could benefit from this amazing "life workout." With their permission I have compiled a small workout in my book designed to help you get as many of the benefits of the Lotte Berk Method as I can. We have photographed several of these core exercises with the help of the vice president, Elisabeth Halfpapp, and her husband, director Fred DeVito. Elisabeth is not only an amazing teacher but also an inspirational woman. I look at her and realize that we can all have the fitness level we want if we are willing to work and balance our lives.

THE 20-MINUTE WORKOUT

I have designed a short workout that you can do when traveling or when you just can't spare the time for a full workout. If the twenty-four hours we get in a day are simply not enough for you but you still want to fit in a workout, here's what to do.

Aerobic training begins when the heart is beating at 65 to 85% of its maximum rate for 12 to 15 minutes. When you're rushed for a workout, I recommend combining your aerobic with your weight training. For the first 5 minutes simply put some music on and lift your legs with bent knees. Your stomach should be engaged the entire time. As you lift your bent leg your feet should be relaxed. Your knees should be above your waist. Let your arms swing freely at first and then you can start with some light weights and do curls at your sides. If you can get outside, run or jog for your first 15 minutes.

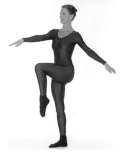

LEG LIFTS. Do at least 100 repetitions, as pictured.

BENT KNEE PUSH-UPS. Get into position with your hands shoulder-width apart and legs hip-width apart, keeping your knees bent and your feet pointed, pulling toward your seat. Do not cross your ankles. With your shoulders down, your head in line, and your chin tucked in, do push-ups, 2 counts

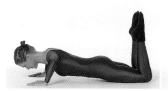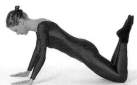

down, 2 counts up (using 1-1,000, 2-1,000 timing). Pull in your abdominals, tucking your pelvis in as if you were pushing your tailbone toward the floor. Work up to 20 repetitions.

BENT-LEG TRICEPS. As pictured, place your hands on the floor at 10 o'clock and 2 o'clock, with thumbs parallel to your body.

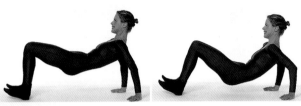

Your knees should be hip-width apart and your feet should be flexed. Raise your hips as high as you can without arching your back. Count slowly to 2 as you lower your body by bending at the elbows. Count to 2 as you raise your body up again. Keep your eyes facing forward. Your range of motion in this exercise won't be great, so keep your shoulders down to make sure your shoulders and neck aren't doing the work your triceps should be doing. Work up to 20 repetitions.

TUMMY CURL. Sit on a mat or towel. Rest your elbows and forearms on the floor, palms down. Tuck your pelvis and your seat underneath your body and pull the abs in, keeping the back of your waist and lower back on the floor. As you slide your arms out, hold onto your outer thighs and pull in abdominals for 30 seconds, then rest on your elbows for a few seconds. Repeat for 30 seconds at a time for about 4 minutes. For advanced tummy work you can work up to keeping your lower back on the floor and releasing your arms and lifting them in the air while you tuck. The further you can pull them closer to your head without losing that tuck with the lower back staying on the floor, the better stretch in your back and strength in your tummy you are attaining.

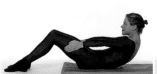
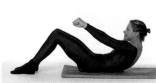
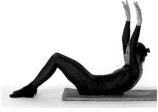

PLIES. Stand an arm's length away from a sturdy chair with your heels together and slightly raised as shown. With your toes at 10 and 2 o'clock, bend at the knees so you lower your body about 5 or 6 inches. Keep your tailbone dropped, your abs sucked in, your shoulders over your hips, and a straight back. Keep this posture; it's very important.

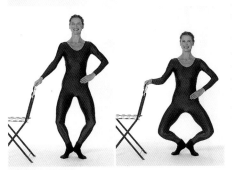

Release and come back up. Do 3 sets of 10 plies. If you have bad knees, skip this exercise.

GRANDE PLIES. These are done in the same basic position as regular plies, but with your legs in a wide stance—heels spread wider than hips. Slowly bend your knees, keeping them directly over your feet, lowering your body until

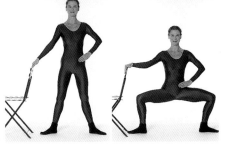

your hips are level with your knees. Count to 2 as you lower and raise your body. Tuck your pelvis in for a more intense exercise. Do 3 sets of 10 plies, resting for a few seconds between each set.

THE ICE SKATER. Fold forearm over forearm. Place arms on the back of a chair. Place your feet hip-width apart, with toes pointed straight ahead. Keep your back perfectly straight (pull in your abs to maintain this posture), and your shoulders down. Raise your right leg up as you rotate your right hip down. Do small, controlled pulses up and down, at least 30 repetitions for each leg. Your thighs should be parallel to the floor and your leg should be straight, toes pointed.

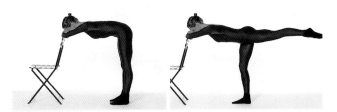

THIGH STRETCH. Sit on your shins with your knees a couple inches apart. Lift your seat off your heels, maintaining a straight back and abs. Relax your elbows slightly, and keep your chin tucked down. For a more advanced stretch, extend your shoulders to the floor.

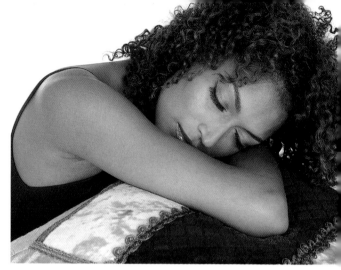

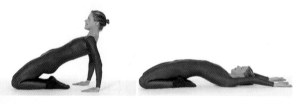

BACK OF LEG STRETCH. Lie on floor with one leg bent, one raised. Wrap a towel around the ball of your flexed foot, as shown. Keep your tailbone and hips pressed flat to the floor as you gently draw your leg back toward your body. If you feel any discomfort, stop pulling. Remember to breathe regularly as you perform this exercise.

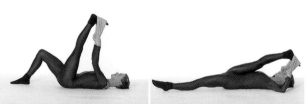

the body relaxers

I know a Body Relaxing Makeover seems like an odd concept, but in our cyber-stressed-out world it could be long overdue for you. I always thought I was an easygoing person, but living in New York City and flying all over the world for work (not to mention the obvious up-keep I need to do as a model) is stressful. I don't pretend to have it bad. Any mother has it much worse. I have enough friends with children to know that juggling a family and a career can take a toll on the most organized of women. That's one of the reasons I began work on this book: to give the overly taxed woman an easy guide to beauty. Well, this makeover is here to help you design your relaxation just as the makeup chapter helps you design your new looks.

Always be on the lookout for scented candles that you love.

I smell everything. You never know where you'll find that perfect scent. If you often buy perfumes that are citrus based, look for citrus-scented candles. Discount department stores often have great deals on closeouts of candles and bath products. Bath and body stores are also great places to find scented candles and aromatherapy oils. You don't have to spend a lot, just be sure you understand what you're buying. Aromatherapy is a wonderful way to learn about scents that affect your moods. If you're stressed, a bath with juniper oil may be just what you need.

Make time every day, even if it's only five minutes, all for you.

Investigate stretching or yoga techniques, depending on your fitness level. Yoga and stretching can contribute to relaxation and mood alteration. A simple routine using basic yoga and orthopedic stretching can make you feel better—and sleep better, too.

Surround yourself with fresh flowers. They don't have to be expensive. One great thing about big "super stores" is that they have large flower departments. On the days you shop, pick up some freshly cut flowers to cheer up your bedroom, bathroom, or kitchen. If you can, grow them in your own garden. Gardening itself can be an effective stress reducer.

Surround yourself with music, or with silence. One of my favorite times is very early in the morning. I love quiet. When I first moved to New York from my small country town I couldn't sleep because of the noise. I started wearing earplugs to bed. I not only loved sleeping with them but I started flying with earplugs as well. When I wear them, there is such a sense of peace for me. Sometimes I don't take them off when I wake up in the morning for an hour or so. I just love having a quiet head. I get teased about it all the time but I don't care. It's my time to have silence, and the rewards are endless.

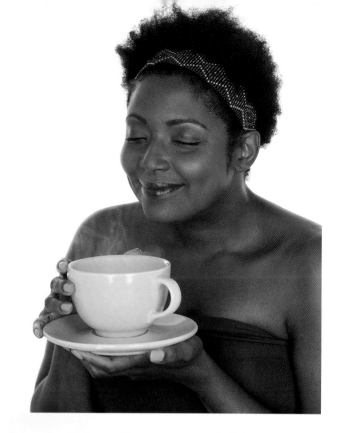

When I'm stressed, I love to slow myself down with a cup of tea. It fills your senses with warmth and whatever aroma you desire.

Get familiar with your body. I want to be in touch with every cell of my body. That's how you know what you want. Many women don't even look at themselves in the mirror—I mean really look—for many different reasons, one being time, another being that they may not see what our society deems "perfect." I'm here to ask you to look.

Cherish your family and friends. If you are lucky enough to have a close relationship with your family then you should enjoy every moment with them. Having a support system is very important.

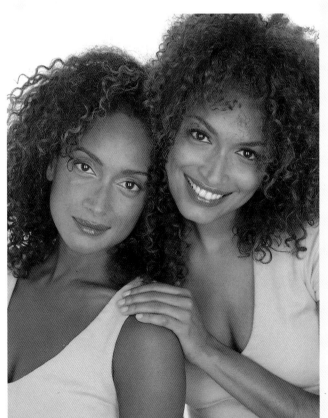

Massage is a great way to relieve stress and get in touch with your body and learn how it works. There are different types of massage (people with phlebitis, high blood pressure, or any other vascular disorders should not receive any type of deep-muscle massage). My favorites are: _Swedish Massage:_ Usually the softest massage, it incorporates kneading, stroking, and tapping to induce relaxation. _Sports Massage:_ Although this employs similar techniques to Swedish massage, it's geared toward sports injuries and the prevention of different ailments associated with sports. Stretching techniques are used to promote flexibility. _Shiatsu:_ This means "finger pressure" in Japanese. It's based on applying pressure to acupressure points to restore and maintain health, relying on energy flows and the effects of pressure blocking.

the energy of beauty

Beauty is about balance. Taking care of the only body you are blessed with is the first part of any beauty routine. Deciding that you want to enhance your beauty or just maintain your body is not something that should be considered shallow. I'm impressed when I see people who really seem to love their bodies. Looking at the structure of your face and body and dealing with the differences that we are all blessed with is important. Knowing that everyone is special (including you) is just the beginning. What you may consider to be a flaw may be the reason others find you unique. So keep this in mind when playing with your makeover. Learn to cherish your unique qualities, for here is where your beauty lies.

Everyone we come in contact with can feel the energy that we emit. We have control of that energy. Every day we can decide how we want to view our lives and the people around us. With regard to beauty, think of the people you know and examine why one appeals to you more than another. Does it have to do with their personal energy or atti-

tude? Many times we are drawn to people simply because their good energy is contagious. They make us feel good when we're around them. Keep these thoughts with you while you make yourself over. Remember that if your energy is bad, no amount of lipstick can cover it up. Choose to be positive, have good energy, don't sweat the small stuff, and watch how a simple makeover can change your life.

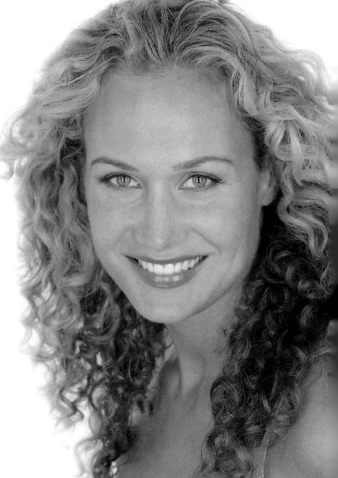

Resources

These are some of my favorite products and services. I've used almost everything that's out there and I will continue to try all the new ones. I'll continue to update this list and provide contact information on my Web site, **www.themakeover.com**. I look forward to chatting with you there!

Moisturizer
L'Oreal FuturE Oil-Free with SPF 15
Mario Badescu Hydra-C Moisturizer

Makeup
Gazzelle Makeup for Women of Color
Laura Mercier Foundation Primer

Concealer/Blush
Laura Mercier Secret Camouflage
L'Oreal Quick Stick Blush

Mascara
L'Oreal Le Grand Curl
Lancôme Extencils

Lip Gloss/Stain
Alchêmy Lip Gloss
Stila Lip Rouge

Makeup Brushes
Laura Mercier and Shu Eumera Synthetic and Natural Hair Brushes
—synthetic flat brush for concealer
—synthetic fine brush for powder under eye
—natural hair angle eye for shadow
—natural hair or synthetic eyeliner brush
—natural hair mid-sized blush brush
—natural hair large-sized powder brush
—natural hair slightly stiff lip brush

Eye Makeup Remover
Lancôme Effacil Eye Makeup Remover

Cleansers
Cetaphil Gentle Cleanser
Mario Badescu Seaweed Cleanser

Hair Products
Phyto Sun Gel Vegan Non–Silicone-Based Hair Gel
J. F. Lazartique Shea Butter for Damaged Hair
Kiehl's Shine & Light Hair Manager

Accessories
Trina Tarantino Jewelry
Suzanne Bennett Accessories

CREDITS

NAIL CARE PRODUCTS
Creative Nail Muscle Top Coat for Weak Nails
Sally Hansen Teflon Tuff Base Coat

FOOT CARE PRODUCTS
The Body Shop Peppermint Foot Scrub
LaCross Manicure and Pedicure Tools

DISCOUNT CLOTHING
Off Fifth from Saks Fifth Avenue
Last Call Neiman Marcus Discount Store

NUTRITION ADVICE
Prescription to Nutritional Healing by James
  Balch, M.D., and Phyliss Balch, CNC
Fit or Fat by Covert Bailey
Weightwatchers International

SKIN CARE CONSULTATION
Dermatology Associates of Atlanta

EXERCISE
The Lotte Berk Method, East Coast

RELAXERS
Rigaud and Lafco Scented and Travel Candles
Bath & Body Works Linen Sprays
Sarafiné Pillow Designs

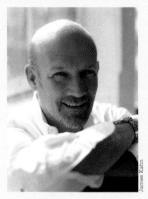

BILL WESTMORELAND has worked in the fashion industry as a makeup artist as well as a photographer for the past twenty years. He recently received his Masters of Fine Arts degree from Norwich University, where he studied photography and filmmaking. Bill lives in New York City and Pennsylvania. Morgen blames him for her obsession with makeup.

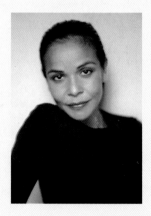

SACHA began her career as a hair stylist at Pippino Buccheri Salon. She is now a freelance stylist working primarily in editorial and advertising. She is Morgen's favorite stylist.